COMPLETE GUIDE TO

SLEEP CARE

Best Practices for a Restful and Happier You

Kiki Ely

chartwell
books

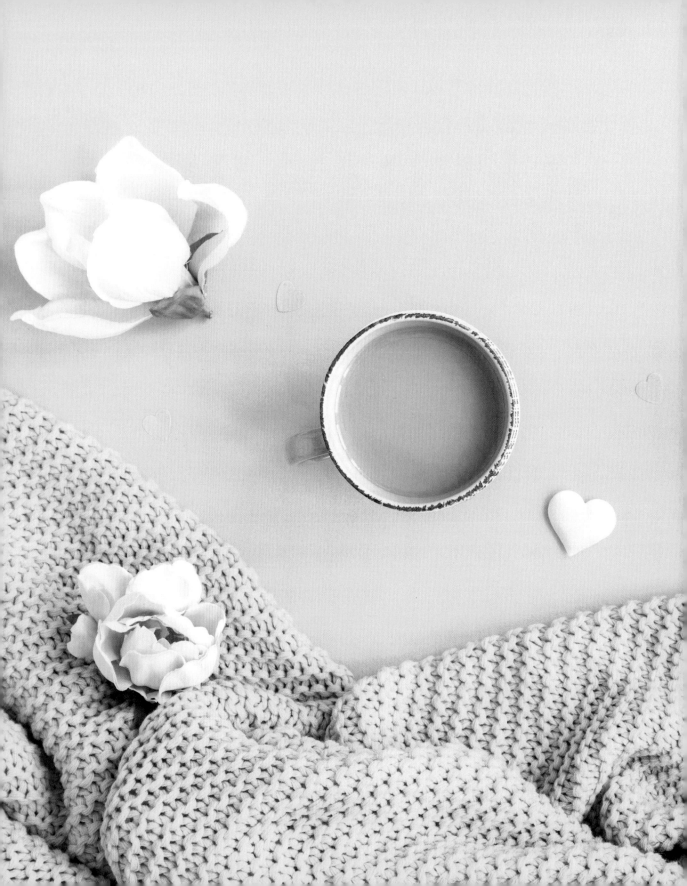

COMPLETE GUIDE TO
SLEEP CARE

Best Practices for a Restful and Happier You

Kiki Ely

chartwell
books

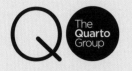

Inspiring | Educating | Creating | Entertaining

Brimming with creative inspiration, how-to projects, and useful information to enrich your everyday life, quarto.com is a favorite destination for those pursuing their interests and passions.

© 2022 Quarto Publishing Group USA Inc.

This edition published in 2022 by Chartwell Books, an imprint of The Quarto Group

142 West 36th Street, 4th Floor New York, NY 10018 USA T (212) 779-4972 F (212) 779-6058

www.Quarto.com

10 9 8 7 6 5 4 3 2

Chartwell titles are also available at discount for retail, wholesale, promotional, and bulk purchase. For details, contact the Special Sales Manager by email at specialsales@quarto.com or by mail at The Quarto Group, Attn: Special Sales Manager, 100 Cummings Center Suite 265D, Beverly, MA 01915, USA.

ISBN: 978-0-7858-4030-5

Library of Congress Control Number: 2021950749

Publisher: Wendy Friedman
Editorial Director: Betina Cochran
Creative Director: Michael Caputo
Editor: Meredith Mennitt
Designer: Sue Boylan
Image credits: Shutterstock

Printed in China

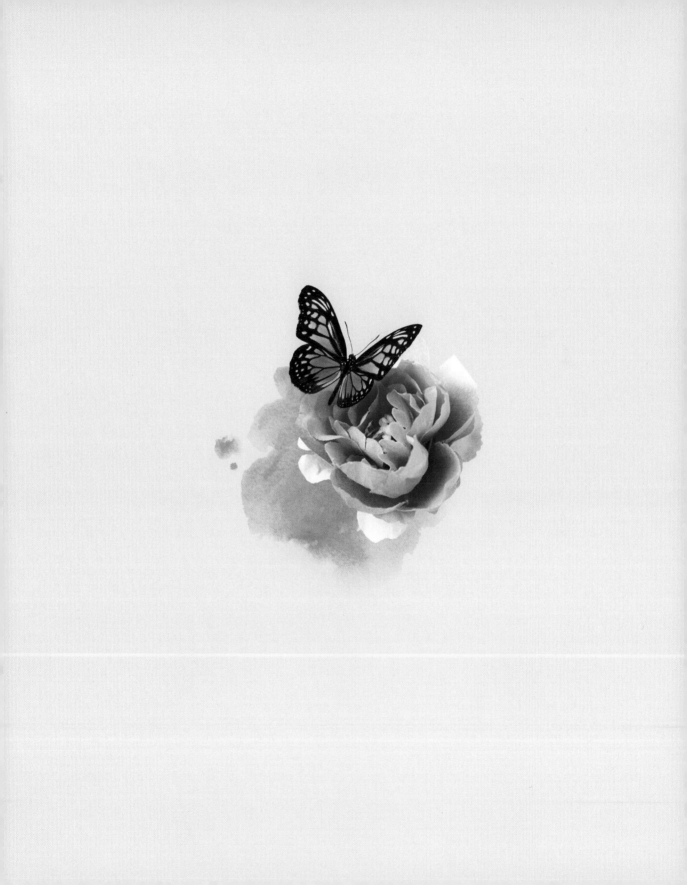

Contents

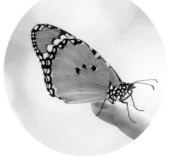

INTRODUCTION — 10

What is Sleep Care?

How to Use This Book

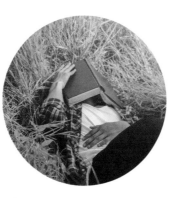

1

THE FOUNDATIONS OF SLEEP

SCIENCE — 16

What Is Sleep?

Two Types of Sleep

The Sleep Cycle

BENEFITS — 20

CIRCADIAN RHYTHM — 22

*Understanding the Roles
of Day and Night*

Rhythm Balancing Exercise

AGE — 26

Sleep Needs Based on Age

*Identify Your Sleep
Schedule Exercise*

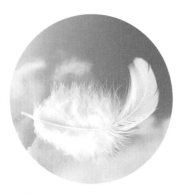

2

SLEEP SANCTUARY

SURROUNDINGS — 32

The Elements of a Sleep Sanctuary

*Dream Your Sanctuary of
Slumber Exercise*

Feng Shui and Your Sleep Sanctuary

*Feng Shui Your Bedroom
Exercise*

SUPPORT — 42

Sleep-Inducing Support

The Perfect Pillow

Mattress Matters

Sleepy Sheets

*Sleepwear for Optimum
Comfort*

*Socks – An Overlooked
Sleep Aid*

*Sleepytime Fabric
Analysis Exercise*

COLOR — 52

The Influence of Color

Using Color to Calm

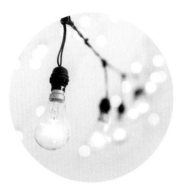

3

GREAT SLEEPS STARTS WITHIN

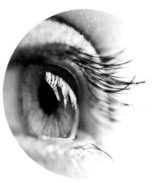

LIGHT — 56

How to Layer the Lighting
in Your Sanctuary

Banishing Blue Light

AIR — 62

Do You Need an Air Purifier?

The Perfect Houseplants for
Healthy Sleep

Identifying Your Ideal Temperature
and Humidity

Prioritizing the Air Around You
Exercise

SCENTS — 66

Essential Oils – The Three You Need

Make Your Own Scented Lotion

Using a Diffuser – Mist or Reed

SOUNDS — 68

Mastering Sound Frequencies

Take a Sound Bath at Home

Create Your Own Soundscape

INNER PEACE — 76

EXERCISE — 78

*Sweat it Out – Great Daytime
Workouts for A Restful Night*

Dance at Home Exercise

EATING & DRINKING — 84

Eating and Drinking for Sleep

Sleepy Food Shopping List

Drinking for Sleep

ROUTINE — 90

Evening Water Ritual –
*Create Your Own
Wind-down Ritual*

Yoga and Meditation

*Intention Setting and the
Phases of the Moon*

Moon Flow Exercise

Breathwork

Breathing for Mindfulness

*Count and Breathe Yourself
to Sleep*

TAMING ANXIETY — 110

How to Get it Out of Your Head
and Onto the Page

Create a Dump Journal

*Drift Off with Thoughts
of Gratitude*

Answer Your Anxiety Exercise

VISUALIZATION — 116

Using Visualization to
Fall Asleep Faster

Empty Room Visualization

Starry Night Visualization

Float Away Visualization

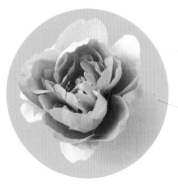

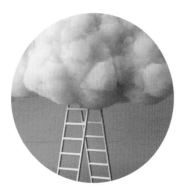

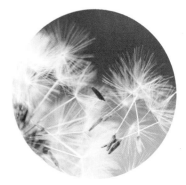

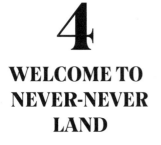

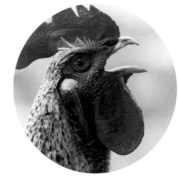

5
RISE AND SHINE WITH INTENTION

LIGHT — 140

Let the Light In

How to Wake Up

The Power of the Slow Start

Your Morning Routine

Wake with Water

Start with Self-Care

Take a Rest Assessment

THE BIG FOUR — 154

Hydration, Affirmation, Movement, and Gratitude

Incorporating Mindfulness and Rest into Your Day

Stop and Breathe

5-minute Anxiety Release

Visualization to Get Present

4
WELCOME TO NEVER-NEVER LAND

DREAMS — 121

The Science of Dreams

Your Subconscious: The Director of the Movies in Your Mind

A Guide to Setting a Dream Intention

Dream Journals

Dream Interpretation

164 — STAY IN TOUCH

166 — THANK YOU & ACKNOWLEDGMENTS

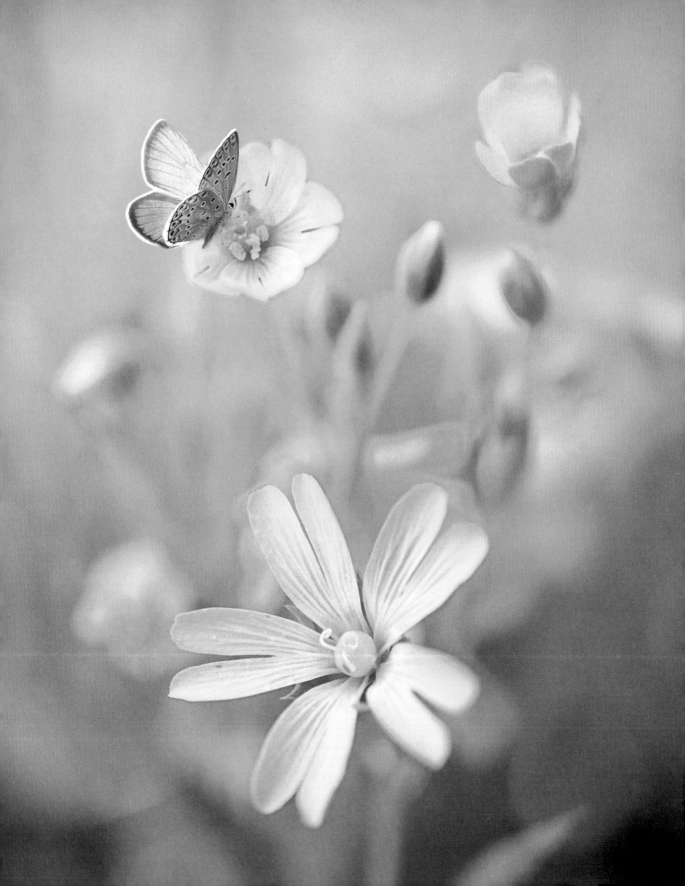

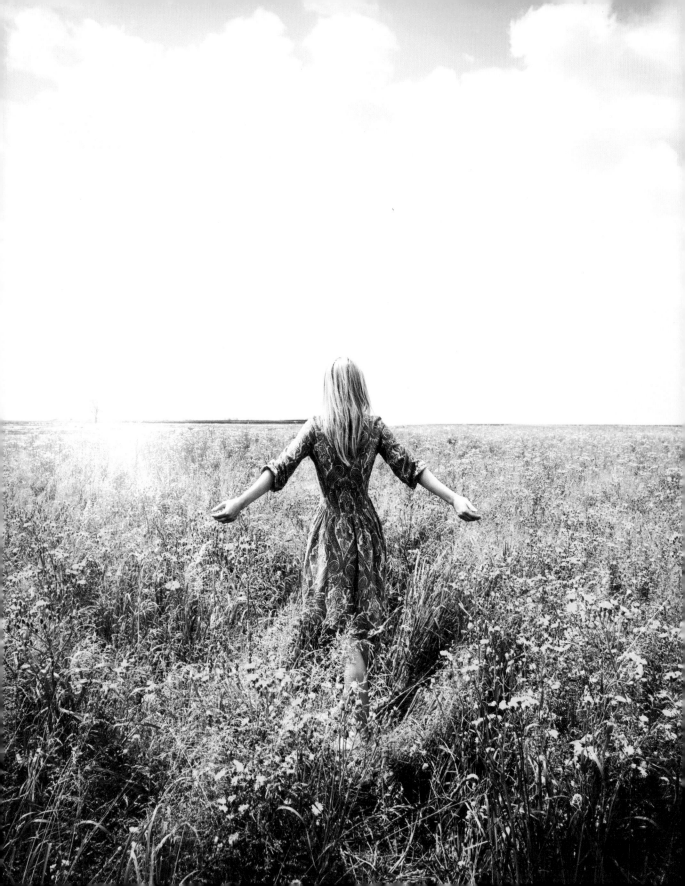

Introduction

Imagine a day where everything is going your way. You feel focused and present. You make decisions with ease. You are aware of your emotions and are able to sustain a feeling of happiness and well-being. You feel energized and calm. You have moments of laughter and moments of connection. You catch a glimpse of yourself in the mirror and you look the way you feel: bright-eyed, joy-filled, and radiant.

—

You might be thinking, *"Yeah, I know that feeling really well! I actually felt that way last week/yesterday/this morning! Life is fantastic!"*

OR

You might be thinking, *"Yeah, right. Stress, indecision, and responsibilities are everywhere. I don't know if I've ever truly felt that way. Life is hard."*

Truth #1: Most people have a train of thought that is closer to the second line of thinking than the first.

Truth #2: The difference between the two modes of thinking is all about mindset, right? Well - sort of. "Mindset" is composed of a bunch of tiny elements, but the foundational element of a positive mindset is (drumroll, please) *quality sleep.*

Not your family. Not your friends. Not a fulfilling job. Not your bank account. Not what you ate for breakfast. Not where you live. Not who you love.

The foundation is sleep.

Simply put: the quality of your sleep is the foundation for the quality of your life.

If that sentence made you panic because you hold the belief that you are "not a good sleeper," stop that mode of thinking right now. Why? Because you have this book. That means that you have countless solutions at your fingertips. You have the ability to retrain - or simply remember - how to sleep.

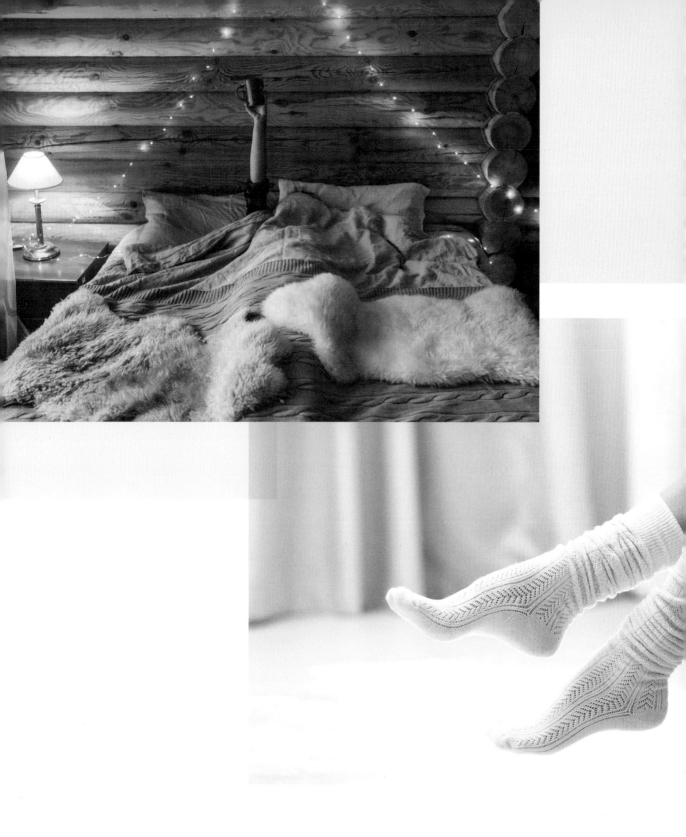

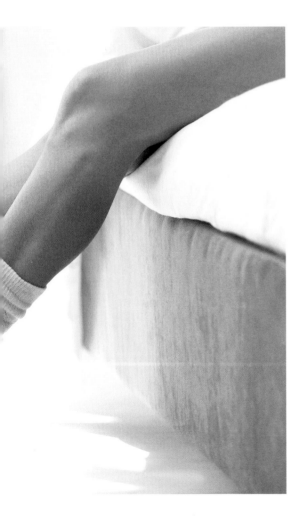

What is Sleep Care?

Sleep care is the creation of habits, the acquisition of knowledge, and the intentional curation of an internal and external environment to facilitate rest.

Most importantly, sleep care is a foundational component of a well-lived life.

How to Use This Book

This book was formatted and organized to allow you to build upon foundational sleep knowledge with each turn of the page.

In addition, this book was also organized in a way that allows you to intuitively use it or to search for something specific using the table of contents.

Feel free to read the book in order from the first page to the last. You can also use the book to address a specific sleeping concern or open the book to any page and start there. This book is a tool for you to use as you see fit.

It was written for you.

However you choose to use this book, my hope is that it enhances your life the same way the knowledge in these pages has enhanced mine.

Love (and lots of light),

KIKI

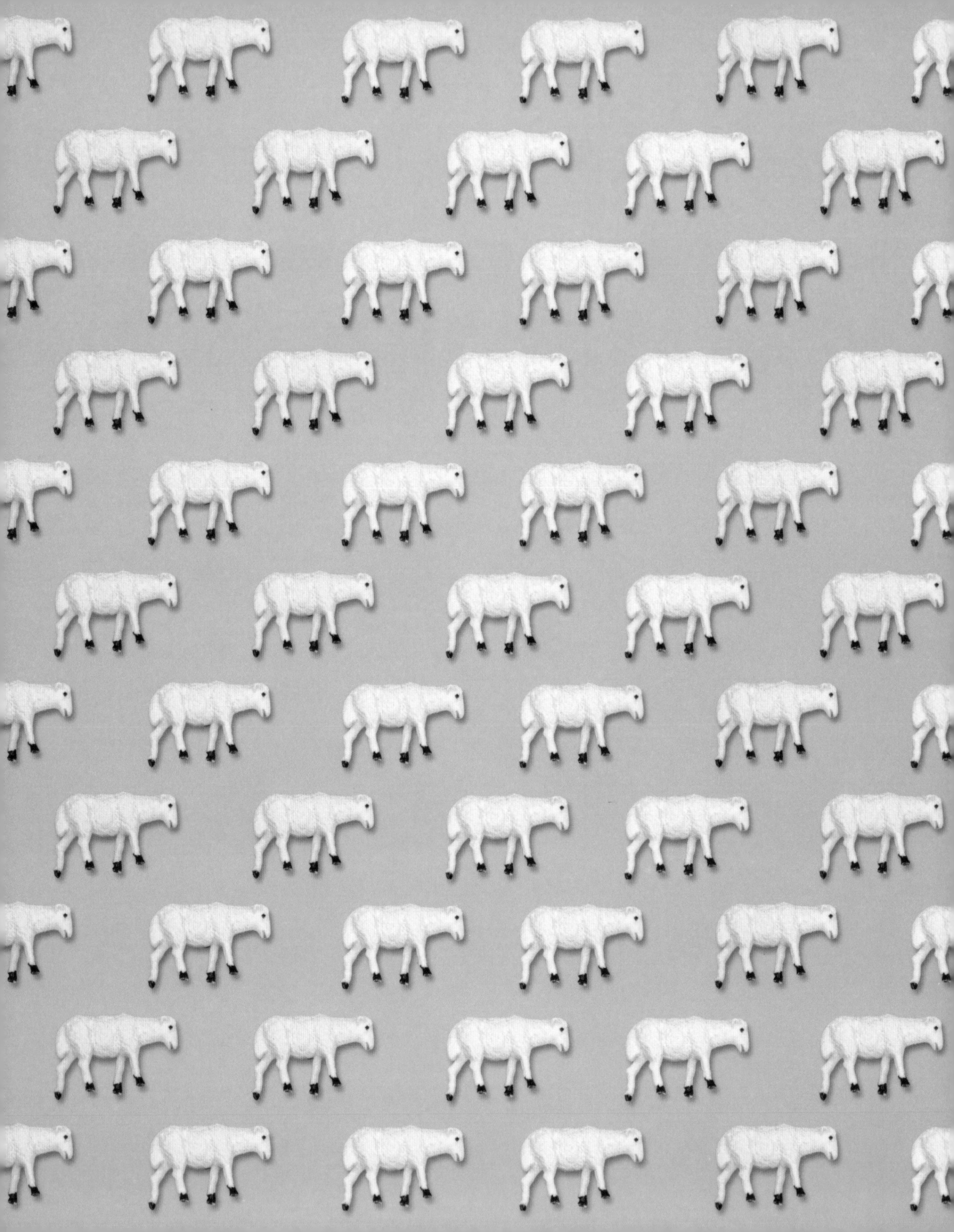

1

THE FOUNDATIONS OF SLEEP

Increase Your Knowledge to Become a Master of Slumber

"It's amazing how lovely common things become, If one only knows how to look at them."

- LOUISA MAY ALCOTT -

The Science of Sleep

For many human beings, the definition of sleep goes something like this:

Sleep [/slēp/] (n): a seemingly simple idea that involves lying down and closing your eyes with the intention of achieving rest that may become increasingly complicated with the addition of racing thoughts, adult responsibilities, and unpredictable environments.

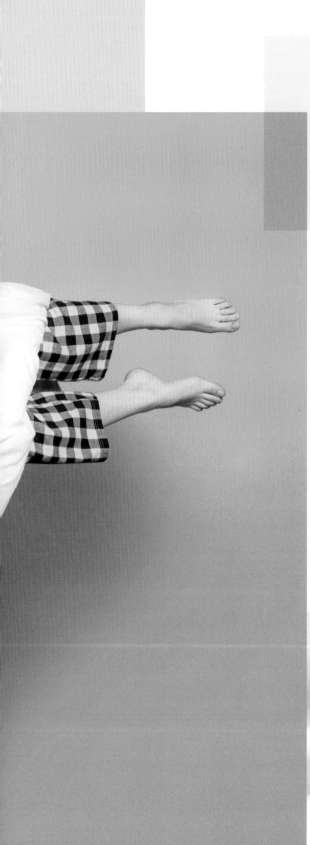

It turns out that sleep is anything but simple. We do not just lie down, fall asleep, and passively allow hours to pass us by. This is what most of humankind believed until sometime around the 1950's when sleep began to be understood scientifically.

—

What Is Sleep?

Sleep is a biological process that involves many components of the brain. Your hypothalamus, brain stem, thalamus, amygdala, and pineal gland are just some of the elements of your brain that have major roles in promoting sleep. During this period of time, your body goes through periods of regeneration and recovery necessary for a healthy physical, mental, and emotional system.

Two Types of Sleep

The type of sleep you experience during a sleep cycle is broken down into two categories: non-REM and REM. REM stands for Rapid Eye Movement. Non-REM sleep consists of three different stages, whereas REM sleep only has one stage.

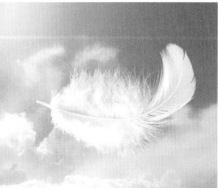

The Sleep Cycle

A typical sleep cycle consists of four stages of sleep. During an average night of sleep, you continue to go through this cycle, as many as four or five times. As the cycle continues to repeat itself, you spend more time in the fourth stage of sleep—REM Sleep—and less time in the third stage of sleep—Non-REM Deep Sleep. If you are sleeping well throughout the night, you will not experience the first stage of the sleep cycle again after the first full cycle has been completed.

It is important to note that the sleep cycle does not always occur sequentially. Typically, you will cycle through the first three stages, then back to the second, and then you'll jump to the fourth. As the cycles go on, you may occasionally skip the third or fourth stage in a given cycle.

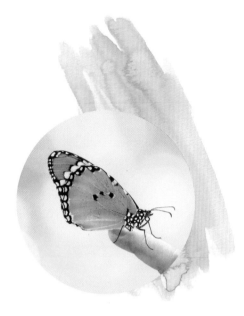

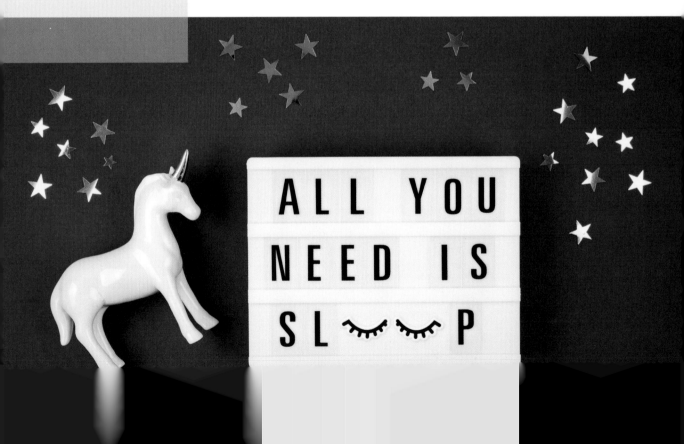

ALL YOU NEED IS SLEEP

THE FIRST STAGE OF SLEEP
Falling Asleep

This Non-REM stage of the sleep cycle is when you transition from wakefulness to sleep. The duration of this stage is usually less than 10 minutes. During this time, your heartbeat, breathing, eye movements, and brain waves begin to slow down. Your muscles will start to relax and you may feel your muscles twitch.

THE SECOND STAGE OF SLEEP
Light Sleep

This is another Non-REM stage of sleep. This light sleep stage lasts around twenty minutes and will repeat throughout the evening as you continue to go through the sleep cycle. About 50% of your total time sleeping each night occurs in this stage. Your heartbeat and breathing slow down further. Your muscles continue to relax more deeply, your body temperature drops, and your eye movements stop. Your brain waves also continue to slow down, but they may be interrupted by short bursts of electrical activity known as sleep spindles. These sleep spindles are thought to assist with the sorting and processing of memories. Scientists believe this is the role of a sleep spindle because an increase in sleep spindle activity occurs the night after someone has learned a lot of new information.

THE THIRD STAGE OF SLEEP
Deep Sleep

The final Non-REM stage of sleep consists of the deep sleep you need to feel fully rested. During this sleep stage, your muscles are fully relaxed and your heartbeat and breath reach their lowest levels. Your brain waves slow down and your brain consolidates things you learned that day. During deep sleep, your body physically repairs itself, releases hormones for bone and muscle health and growth, and strengthens your immunity.

THE FOURTH STAGE OF SLEEP
Dream Sleep

During this stage of REM sleep, your eyes move from side to side while your eyes are closed. This cycle occurs about 90 minutes after falling asleep and continues to repeat throughout the night. Your heart, blood pressure, breathing, and brain waves come close to matching their waking levels. Your arm and leg muscles are paralyzed to keep you safe while you dream. Though dreaming can occur in other stages of sleep, most dreams occur during the REM stage. As you age, your REM cycles become shorter.

The Benefits of Sleep

Sleep is necessary for your health, regeneration, focus, energy, and memory. It is connected to your mood, sense of well-being, and overall satisfaction. It impacts your appetite, desires, and mindset. When you do not get a good night of rest, you may feel distracted, sluggish, on edge, or struggle to make it through the day.

The quality of your physical health is directly linked to the quality of your sleep. The risk of seizures, headaches, and high blood pressure increase when you do not get enough sleep. Good sleep habits are correlated with a healthier heart. Your immune system works less efficiently when you are sleep-deprived, which increases your likelihood of falling ill. Sleep is a necessary component for your body to adequately heal physical injuries. For optimum physical regeneration, it is imperative to enter deep sleep, or the third stage of sleep.

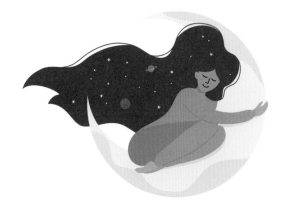

Your weight is another element of physical health that is impacted by sleep. Your body needs to enter deep sleep for your blood sugar to regulate itself. While in deep sleep, your glucose levels drop, allowing your body to rest and calibrate its blood sugar needs. A lack of sleep also causes the hormones that regulate your appetite to shift, which may lead you to overeating. Additionally, without the energy that sleep provides, you may be less motivated or capable to exercise and more motivated to grab a high-sugar snack, which may also lead to weight gain.

Physical attractiveness is linked to physical health. If you do not allow yourself enough time to physically regenerate during sleep, you may notice that your appearance is negatively impacted. Your eyes may appear sunken or they might lose a bit of the brightness or spark, appearing flat. You might develop dark under eye circles. Your face may appear hollow and your skin might seem lackluster.

Brain function and efficiency are also inextricably linked with sleep. If you seek to concentrate and learn something new, desire to strengthen your memory, and want to keep your brain free and clear of toxins, then sleep is necessary. Sleep has a direct impact on "brain plasticity," which is your brain's ability to incorporate and integrate the input it receives. When you sleep well, it is easier for you to learn and to remember. A poor night of sleep can negatively impact your ability to retain information. For your brain to utilize proper problem-solving, decision-making, and even to access its source of creativity you need quality sleep. The brain experiences the greatest benefits during the REM stage of sleep.

Sleep can have an impact on your mood, as well. Your brain needs sleep to process, organize, and recognize emotions. When the brain does not have the time to do this, it can lead to depression, anxiety, panic attacks, or other mood disorders. Short of a mood disorder, a poor night of sleep can impact your ability to control and regulate your daily emotions. Dreams, which occur most frequently during REM sleep, are also theorized to assist with the processing of emotions.

Sleep impacts your physical, emotional, and mental health at a fundamental level. To achieve your highest potential in life—and to live your most fulfilling life—you must prioritize a healthy sleep life.

Your Circadian Rhythm

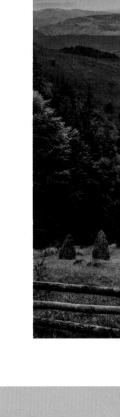

Your Circadian Rhythm

Your circadian rhythm is a twenty-four-hour cycle connected to your internal clock that regulates important processes for your body, such as appetite, hormones, and sleep. You can think of your circadian rhythm as a piece of your internal programming connected to a teeny-tiny clock inside of your brain that, when calibrated correctly, keeps all of the systems in your body running at the appropriate time. This teeny-tiny clock is located in the suprachiasmatic nucleus, or SCN, which is found in the hypothalamus in your brain. This internal clock is calibrated using a variety of factors, but the most influential is light. Your body's internal clock sets itself by recognizing the difference between light and darkness from signals sent to your brain by your eyes.

When your circadian rhythm is synced correctly, lightness—or daylight—causes your body to enter an energetic state by releasing a hormone known as cortisol. On the flip side, darkness—or nighttime—causes your body to release melatonin, a hormone that aids in sleep. When your circadian rhythm is off, you may not be able to fall asleep or stay asleep, and you may feel disoriented or sluggish during the day.

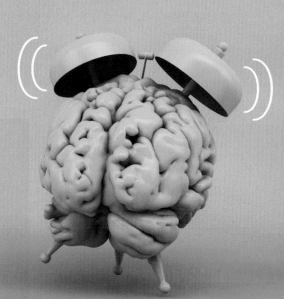

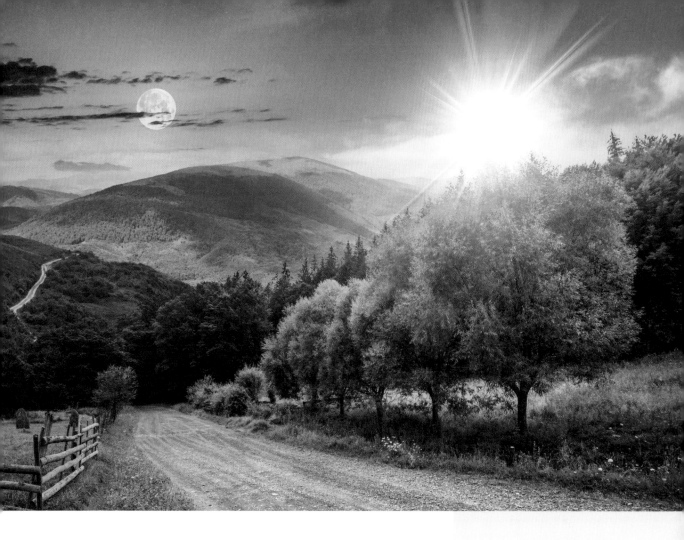

Understanding the Roles of Day and Night

Before the introduction of electricity, people would use the sun as their timepiece. The day would begin with the rising of the sun and would wind down with the setting of the sun. This meant that the circadian rhythms of human beings were naturally in alignment with the timing of the day and the night.

Today's modern lifestyle introduces a series of complications when calibrating your internal clock. The first is the introduction of electricity. Due to electricity, sources of artificial light are found everywhere; your eyes can now absorb light before sunrise and after sunset. The next is the introduction of technology. The light from your screens - television, computer, tablet, or cell phone - is being interpreted as natural light by your brain, further confusing your internal clock. The final complication is a sedentary lifestyle. Many people do not interact with natural light during the day. They may leave their home to work before the sun rises and arrive home after the sun has set. They may stay indoors for the entire day. This further confuses the internal clock, as it now bases its timing of day and night solely on artificial light.

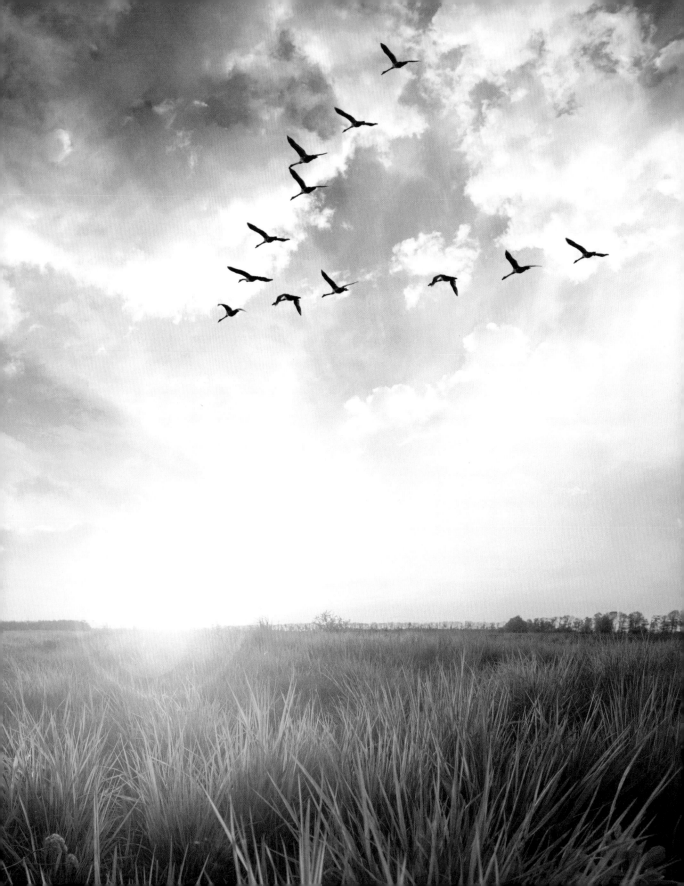

Circadian Rhythm Balancing Exercise

If your circadian rhythm is out of calibration, you can experience drowsiness and fatigue during the day and an inability to fall asleep and stay asleep at night. You can reset your circadian rhythm by completing the following exercise. You may find this exercise is balancing for you because it creates a routine that gets you outside to breathe in fresh air and connect with nature. If you enjoy it, you can turn this exercise into a part of your daily life.

1. **Choose your duration.** Commit to a period of time between three and fourteen consecutive days. The longer you incorporate this practice, the more consistent and predictable your circadian rhythm will become.

2. **Determine the time for sunrise and sunset.** Look up the timing for sunrise and sunset. You can do this by using the internet or checking the local paper.

3. **Set your schedule.** For each day of the exercise, set an alarm or a reminder on your phone (you can use your phone's calendar app to do this), for ten minutes before sunrise and sunset.

4. **Rise with the sun.** When your morning alarm goes off, get up and go outside. Find a comfortable position, sitting or standing, and watch the sunrise. Turn your face towards the sun. Sit outside for ten minutes after the sun has risen.

5. **Screens disappear when the sun sets.** When your evening alarm goes off, turn off all screens in your home. Turn off televisions, computers, phone, or any screen that emits light. For greater impact, you can also dim or minimize the other sources of artificial light in your home. Go outside, turn your face towards the sun, and watch the sunset. Sit outside for 10 minutes after the sun has set.

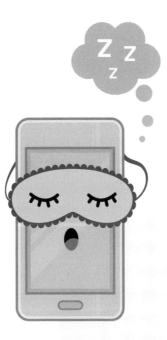

6. **Repeat.** Do this each day for the time period you identified in step one.

7. **Bonus points.** If you want to make this exercise even more effective, do not take a nap while you are resetting your internal clock. Also, aim to go to bed around the same time each night to deeply calibrate your body.

MODIFICATION:

If you live in an area with inclement weather or an area where daylight hours are impacted (due to living in a very northern or southern region of the world), the previous exercise can still benefit you. Instead of looking up the time for sunrise and sunset each day, choose a consistent waking time and decompression time and commit to them. Use a sun lamp or mood lamp, which can be purchased online, in lieu of the sunrise. When you wake up at your chosen time, sit in front of the lamp for 10 minutes. This creates the illusion of sunlight for your internal clock. When your decompression alarm (in lieu of a sunset alarm) goes off, turn off all of the screens in your home and minimize your sources of artificial light. Repeat this for a minimum of three days.

Sleep Needs Based on Age

The average adult needs between seven and nine hours of quality sleep each night to function well. It can be difficult for young adults and seniors to get this amount of sleep each night. Young adults are more prone to suffer from depression which negatively impacts the ability to sleep. They may also make lifestyle choices, like staying up late to be with friends, that cut into the amount of quality sleep they receive each night. Seniors naturally begin to cycle through deep sleep stages at lower frequencies as they age. Some medications they take can also disrupt their sleep cycle. This means both young adults and seniors may benefit from a daily nap to help with any sleep deficit they may experience.

—

A teenager needs about an hour more of quality sleep a night than an adult, so a teen should aim for eight and ten hours of sleep a night. Additionally, teens have a circadian rhythm that operates differently than adults. Their internal clock tells them to go to sleep after 11 p.m. and to wake up later in the day. As the modern school schedule is not in alignment with a teenager's natural sleep needs, a teen can combat their internal clock by sticking to a regimented sleeping schedule that involves going to sleep earlier than their body initially tells them to.

Studies have determined that women need approximately twenty minutes more sleep each night than men do. Though the reason behind this has not been fully understood, there is a theory that because women tend to be busier and more prone to multitasking that their brains may need more time to recuperate from the day's exertion.

In select cases, some adults only need 4–5 hours of sleep to function properly, but this is far from the norm. To determine if you fall into this category, take note of how you feel the day or days after a shorter night of sleep. If you feel a bit groggy, sleepy, or find yourself reaching for quick energy fixes like caffeine and sugar, then you are not sufficiently rested on this amount of sleep. If, however, you feel great, your mood is stable, and you have plenty of energy, you may be one of the few (lucky!) individuals who have the ability to function at their highest on less sleep.

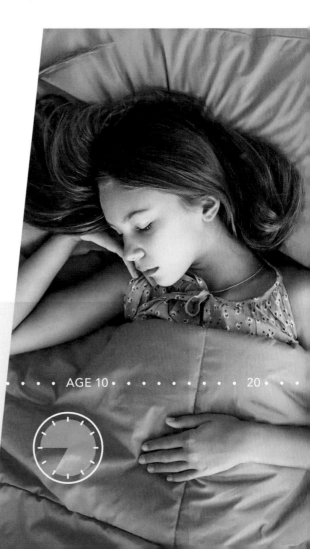

AGE 10 · · · · · · · · · · 20 · · · ·

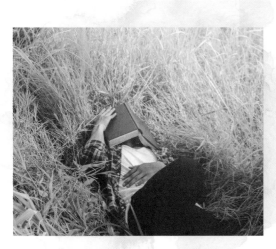

To Nap or Not to Nap

A nap—as long as it is twenty minutes or less and timed correctly—can be very beneficial to making up for a poor night's rest. When you nap for longer than twenty minutes, your body enters a deeper phase of sleep, which makes it harder to wake up and you may experience a groggy feeling. Additionally, a late afternoon nap can negatively impact your ability to fall asleep and stay asleep at night. Aim for a twenty minute nap that happens sometime before 3 p.m.

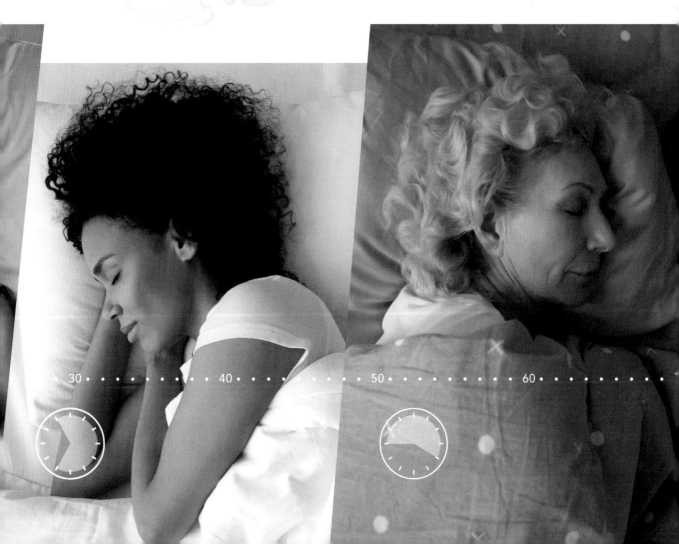

Identify Your Sleep Schedule Exercise

Keeping a regular sleep routine is the first step to ensuring you receive quality sleep.

① **Pick Your Week.** Look at your calendar and upcoming obligations. Find a week that you can commit to a consistent sleep schedule. A consistent sleep schedule involves waking up and going to sleep at the same time each day.

② **Incorporate Your Partner.** If you share a bed with a partner, make sure to inform them of your goal. This way, they can be considerate with their sleep timing throughout the duration of this exercise. Even better if they decide to participate with you!

③ **Identify Your Schedule.** Using the following chart, find your recommended amount of sleep for optimum health. Then determine what time you will go to sleep each night and wake each morning to allow enough time for quality sleep.

AGE	SLEEP NEEDED
13–18	8–10 hours
18–65	7–9 hours
65+	7–8 hours

④ **Use Accountability Alarms.** Set an alarm each day for your waking time and for twenty minutes before your bedtime. The twenty-minute window is to allow you enough time to prepare for bed and wind down.

⑤ **Check in Morning, Noon, and Night.** Each morning after you wake, each day at lunch, and each evening before bed, take note of your energy levels. If your energy is high in the morning, moderately high midday, and a bit lower at night, then you are getting quality sleep.

⑥ **Adjust Accordingly.** If you notice that your energy levels have not yet improved, do not worry. It takes a few days for the body to calibrate to good sleep. If, after a few days, your energy levels have not improved, make your bedtime thirty minutes earlier than originally scheduled.

⑦ **Identify Your Ideal Schedule – Take More Time if You Need It.** At the end of the week, you should have a relatively good idea as to your optimum sleep schedule. If you still feel unsure, just do it again! You can try to adjust your waking and sleeping times slightly until you find a rhythm that works for you.

Note: If you are currently pregnant or you have a baby (or more than one baby!), then this exercise can be modified. You can still set a sleeping and waking time, but the time in between will be a bit more unpredictable. Pregnant women deal with many hormonal and physical changes that make staying asleep and reaching levels of deep sleep more difficult. Women with babies can also set a sleeping and waking time, but the behavior of the baby (feeding times, crying, etc.) can be unpredictable and interrupt deep sleep. For pregnant women or mothers of babies, this exercise is still helpful in establishing a sleep schedule. Be gentle with yourself if you find that you cannot sleep—or stay in bed—between your set times.

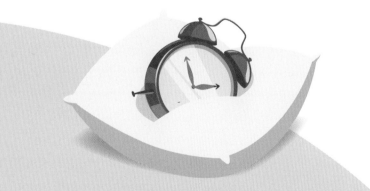

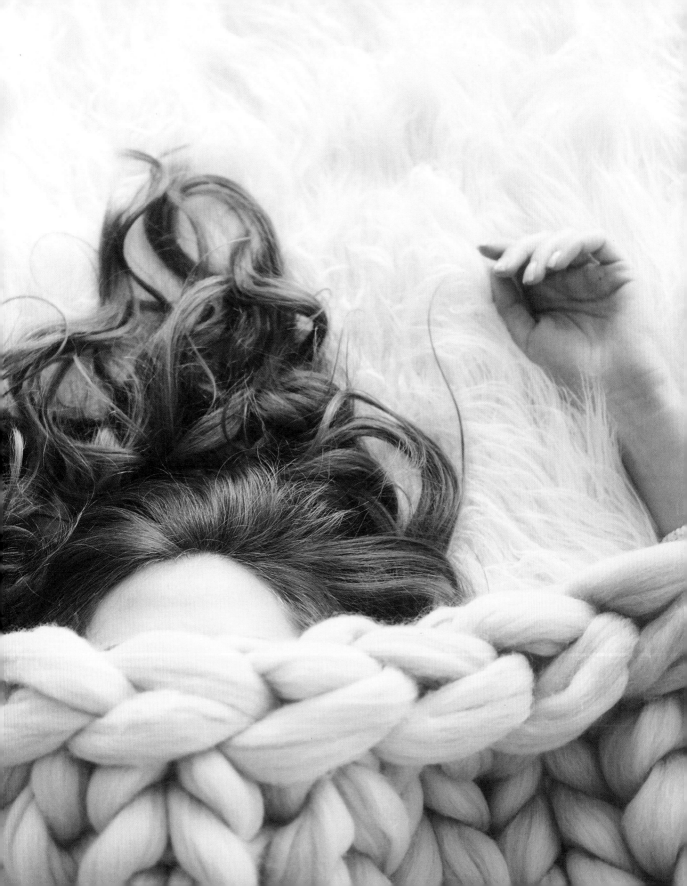

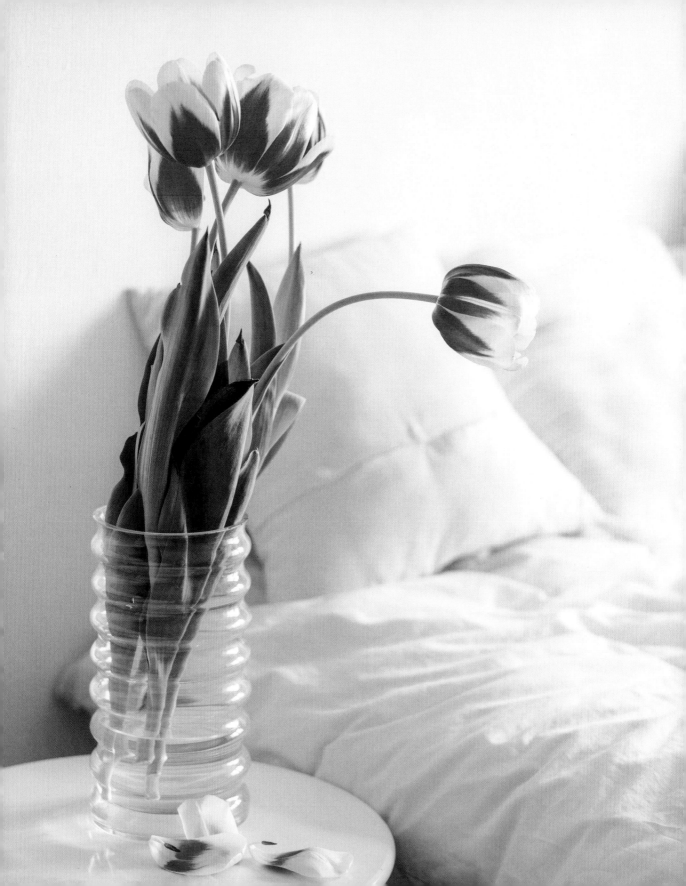

2

SLEEP SANCTUARY

How to Consciously Curate Your
Surroundings and Stimuli to Promote Rest

"Peace at home, peace in the world."
- MUSTAFA KEMAL ATATÜRK -

Surroundings for Sleep

If I were to ask you: *How are you feeling?* You would likely check in with yourself and think something like: *Hmm. I guess I feel a little bit distracted. I'm kind of happy. Now that I think about it, I'm also slightly overwhelmed.*

Imagine if instead you thought: *I feel a little bit distracted because there is quite a lot going on around me right now. I can see piles of things I have to wash and bills I have to pay. I also hear noise from a television in the background. I guess that's making it difficult for me to collect my thoughts. I'm kind of happy because someone has taken the time to ask me how I am feeling, and that makes me feel cared for. Perhaps I'm slightly overwhelmed because the clutter around me reminds me of everything I have not completed.*

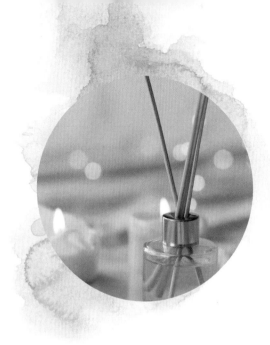

—

What is the difference between the two modes of thinking? The first is completely focused on what is going on inside of you and the second *takes into account* what is going on outside of you.

Your environment has a tremendous impact on your state of mind. As an example of this, imagine yourself in the following two settings:

Setting #1: You go to see your favorite band play a sold out show. You are surrounded by colored lights, countless people, and enveloped by the sound of the music. You feel alive, excited, and full of energy!

Setting #2: You go to a spa for a massage. You enter a treatment room with soft lighting, neutral colors, and soothing nature sounds. You feel calm, present, and completely relaxed.

Both of these environments are wonderful in their own right, and both environments can contribute to your happiness. However, one environment promotes happiness at a high-energy level and the other promotes joy at a more tranquil frequency.

The environment in which you rest should be entirely focused on creating a joyful and tranquil experience. This better facilitates being able to fall asleep and stay asleep. All high-energy creating stimuli should be banned from your bedroom.

Yes, banned.

Why? Because the average human spends twenty-six years sleeping and seven years trying to sleep. If that didn't make your jaw drop, read it again. You spend around a third of your life in bed. If you do not optimize your bed and the area surrounding it, you are settling for a below average rest and rejuvenation experience. You—based on the fact that you are taking the time to read this book—are not someone who settles for a below average life experience.

This chapter will assist you with identifying things you can improve in your bedroom today. It will also help you understand how small changes can have a significant impact on the quality of your sleep. Most importantly, it will ensure that you are not one of the millions of people who have settled for a below average sleep experience. You deserve so much more than that—and you know it.

The Elements of a Sleep Sanctuary

To navigate this chapter, it is important that you first understand the basic elements that make up a sleep sanctuary.

—

Imagine your ideal sleep space in vivid detail. It is necessary to do this before moving forward in the chapter so that you are in alignment with what you naturally gravitate towards before being influenced by any suggestions.

Repeat this exercise at the end of the chapter after absorbing all of the information and suggestions contained within it to fully refine your vision and put it into action.

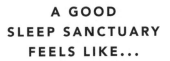

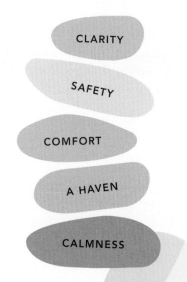

A GOOD
SLEEP SANCTUARY
FEELS LIKE...

CLARITY

SAFETY

COMFORT

A HAVEN

CALMNESS

A GOOD SLEEP SANCTUARY DOES NOT HAVE...

Clutter

Too much stuff or oversized furniture

Any work related materials

Bright lighting and poor air quality

Uncomfortable fabrics

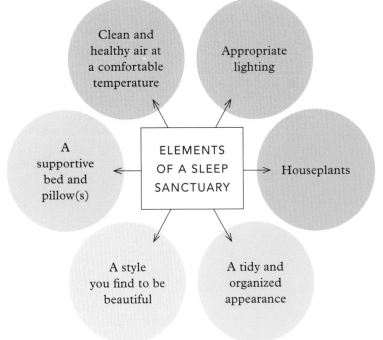

ELEMENTS OF A SLEEP SANCTUARY

Clean and healthy air at a comfortable temperature

Appropriate lighting

A supportive bed and pillow(s)

Houseplants

A style you find to be beautiful

A tidy and organized appearance

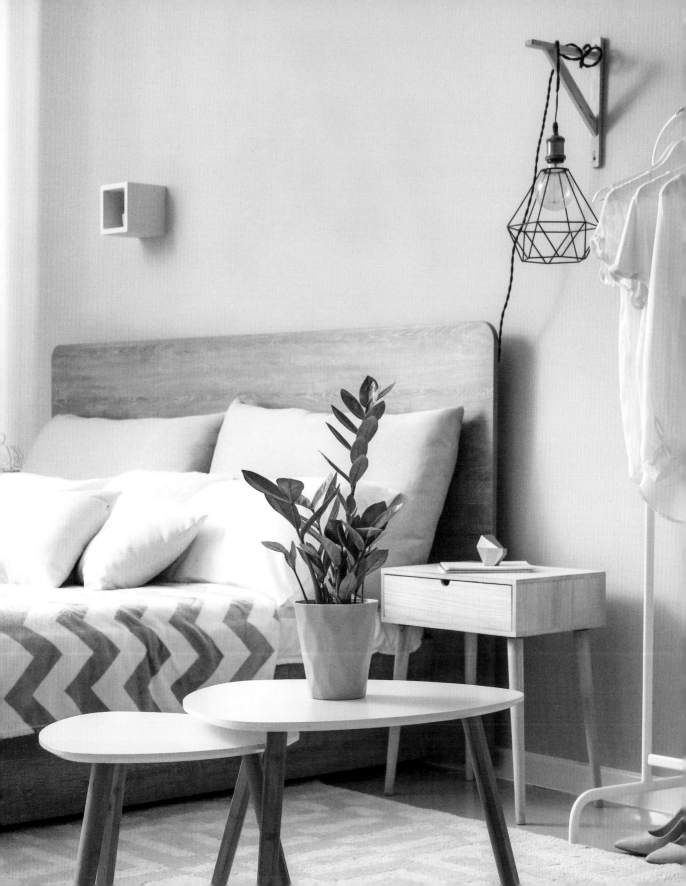

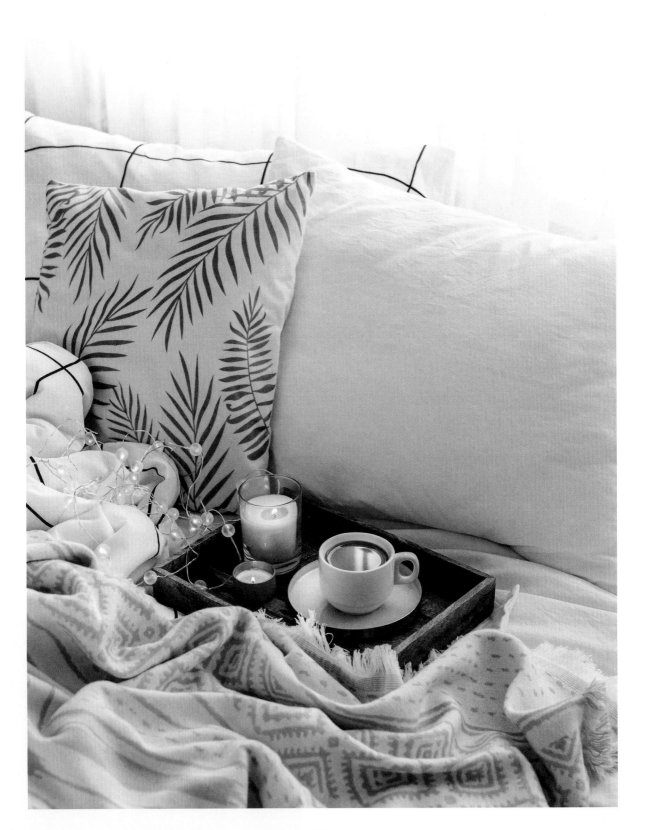

Dream Your Sanctuary of Slumber Exercise

The first step to creating the sleep sanctuary of your dreams is to clearly visualize the space.

Visualization is simply:
• Identifying what you want to see.
• Imagining it.

If you are concerned that you are not very imaginative, it will not hinder your results in this exercise. You will be guided to focus on your five senses to activate your imagination.

The following exercise will help you plan your perfect rest-filled room.

1 Sit somewhere comfortable and quiet and close your eyes. Breathe deeply until you feel calm. Once you are calm and present, move onto the next step.

2 Think of yourself standing in your bedroom with all of the furniture removed and all of the walls bare. It is a blank canvas.

3 You will start by engaging your sense of sight. Visualize a beautiful and comfortable bed in the room. Take notice of what the bed looks like. Imagine the frame, the comforter, the pillows, and the sheets. Notice where it is placed in the room. If something doesn't come in clearly for you right away, take your time. Continue to breathe. Keep visualizing the bed. Once it is in clear view, move onto the next step.

4 You will now engage your sense of touch. Visualize yourself walking up to the bed, pulling the covers back, and lying down. Imagine that the bed you are lying on is the most comfortable bed you have ever been in. Feel the mattress against your body and the pillow cradling your head and neck. Feel the fabric of the sheets and the weight of the comforter. Once you have felt the comfort surrounding you, move onto the next step.

5 You will now engage your sense of taste. Visualize a bedside table. On it sits a soothing and hydrating beverage in a lovely glass or cozy mug. Imagine any beverage you like. Visualize yourself sitting up in bed and slowly drinking the beverage. Taste each sip of the beverage you chose. Once you have done this, move onto the next step.

6 You will now engage your sense of smell. Visualize yourself inhaling the scent of the beverage in your cup. Take note of the nuances in the smell. Now breathe in the scent of your room. Imagine that you are smelling the most calming and lovely scent. You now notice that this scent is coming from your bedside table. Visualize a candle, a diffuser, or essential oils sitting on top of the table. Once you have done this, move onto the next step.

7 You will now engage your sense of sound. Visualize yourself closing your eyes and listening. You hear the most relaxing and soothing sound you can imagine. It might be silence or light music or nature sounds. Once you have done this, open your eyes.

8 Write down the specifics of your bed, bedside table, calming beverage, the scents in your sanctuary, and what you heard. Keep this in a safe place because you will revisit it at the end of the chapter.

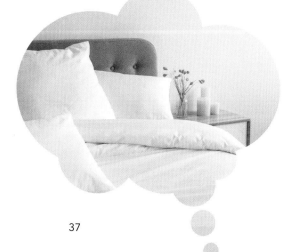

Feng Shui and Your Sleep Sanctuary

Feng shui is an interior design philosophy that is based on the belief that the flow of energy within a space can be influenced by the arrangement and placement of objects within that space. The art of feng shui is based on the belief that life energy—or chi—can be encouraged to flow freely or can become blocked based on the arrangement of objects in your home. This ancient practice is used today by many interior designers, architects, energy workers, and everyday people.

If the idea of energy being connected to objects in a room seems a little far-fetched to you, that doesn't mean that you should disregard feng shui. The practice of feng shui creates undeniable balance in a room which results in a sense of calmness and peace. The room will have good "flow"—meaning that the placement of items makes sense, you can move easily about the room, and you feel good in the space.

Feng shui practitioners utilize something called a bagua map. The bagua map is broken into nine different sections, all associated with different colors, natural elements, shapes, and facets of life.

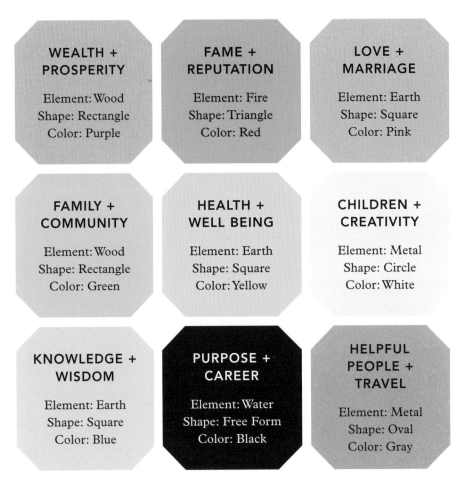

WEALTH + PROSPERITY

Element: Wood
Shape: Rectangle
Color: Purple

FAME + REPUTATION

Element: Fire
Shape: Triangle
Color: Red

LOVE + MARRIAGE

Element: Earth
Shape: Square
Color: Pink

FAMILY + COMMUNITY

Element: Wood
Shape: Rectangle
Color: Green

HEALTH + WELL BEING

Element: Earth
Shape: Square
Color: Yellow

CHILDREN + CREATIVITY

Element: Metal
Shape: Circle
Color: White

KNOWLEDGE + WISDOM

Element: Earth
Shape: Square
Color: Blue

PURPOSE + CAREER

Element: Water
Shape: Free Form
Color: Black

HELPFUL PEOPLE + TRAVEL

Element: Metal
Shape: Oval
Color: Gray

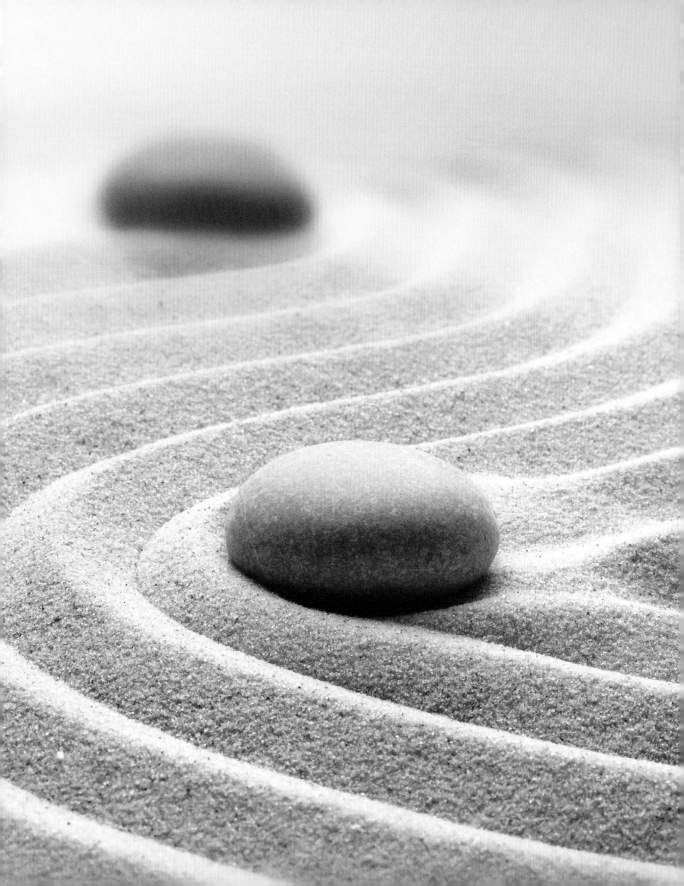

Feng Shui Your Bedroom Exercise

The following exercise will help you implement the tenets of feng shui in your bedroom. This will increase a feeling of balance, calmness, and positive energy.

(1) Locate the main entry door to your room and line it up with the bottom of your bagua map. Imagine the bagua map overlaying the floor of your bedroom as if you were looking down from the sky into your room. To be even more thorough, you can print out or draw a floorplan of your bedroom and then draw an evenly spaced 3x3 grid, creating the nine bagua map sections, over the floorplan to determine which area of your bedroom falls into each area of the bagua map.

(2) Identify three topics on the bagua map that you would like to improve in your life. If you are looking for a new job or are dissatisfied with your work, you might want to focus on the "Purpose and Career" section of the map. If you have a financial goal in mind, you may want to focus on the "Wealth and Prosperity" section of the map. If you would like to improve your marriage or find a spouse, you would focus on the "Love and Marriage" section on the map.

(3) Identify the three areas you have selected on the map in your bedroom. You will be arranging these three areas to bring them into alignment with the suggestions on the bagua map.

(4) Identify the elements on the bagua map that you are going to incorporate into those areas of your bedroom. For example: if you had selected "Family and Community" as one of your goals in Step 2, you would incorporate items that are connected to the wood element, are rectangular in shape, and/or are green. Not every item in this area needs to fit this criteria. Also, a singular item does not need to satisfy all criteria, but an item can.

For example: this area might be a spot where you have a cozy blue chair. This is not wood, rectangular, or green. It can still stay in this area if you choose. You might place a wooden side table next to the chair. If this table is rectangular, it will satisfy the wood and rectangle elements.

If it is round, it will satisfy the wood element. You might place a framed photo of a forest on the wall above the chair. The frame might be made of wood, rectangular in shape, and the painting is of a lush green forest. This item would satisfy the wood, rectangle, and green elements.

(5) Repeat this for each area in your bedroom that you identified on your bagua map. If you enjoy the sense of balance this brings to your space, you can incorporate other areas of the bagua map until you have addressed all nine sections.

Note: if you find that feng shui-ing your bedroom was therapeutic, don't stop there! You can feng shui any room in your home for a more peaceful and serene living experience. Here's a suggestion on the next place to feng shui: your napping spot. Many people nap in a chair or on a couch that they love. Incorporate the above tenets into your napping spot for an increased feeling of tranquility.

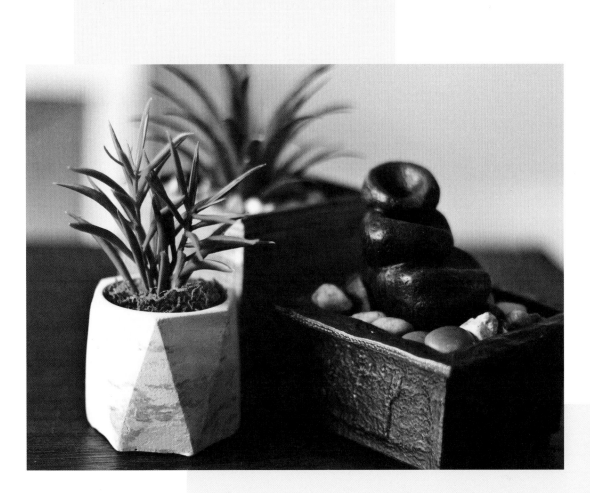

Suggested Items for Different Elements

You can get creative when choosing items to satisfy different elements, shapes, and colors. Colors and shapes are something you are likely quite familiar with at this point in your life, but you may not be as familiar with the elements. Here are some suggestions to help get you started.

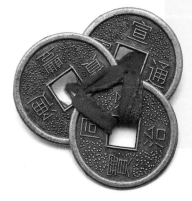

Earth: geodes, clay goods, a potted plant in soil
Water: a water feature, a painting of a lake, a photo of the beach
Metal: a silver tray, a metal sculpture, beautiful jewelry
Fire: candles, a photo of the sun, a space heater
Wood: wooden furniture, art with trees in it, wooden picture frames

Sleep-Inducing Support

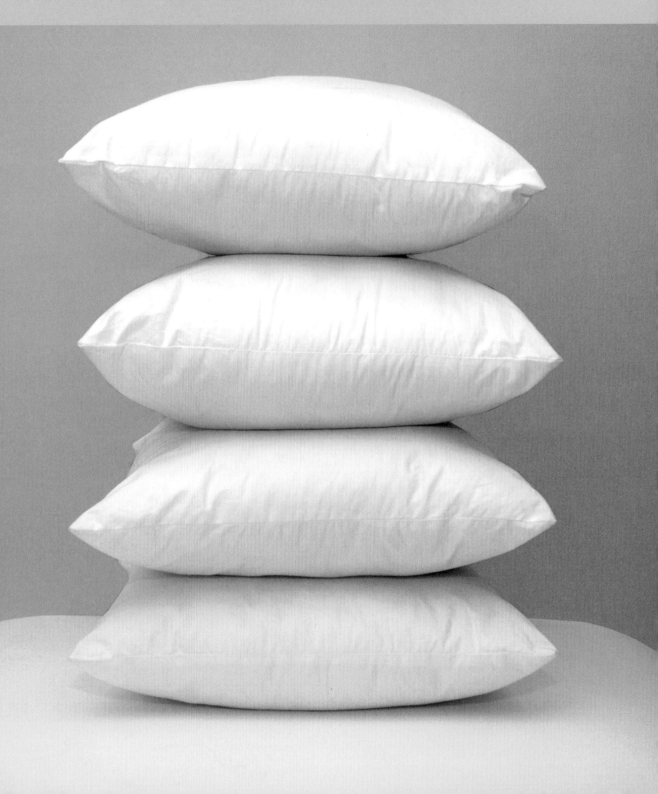

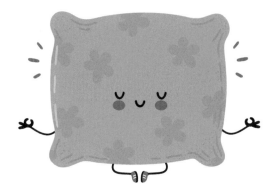

While you sleep, your senses are almost completely disengaged. You are, however, still experiencing the sense of touch. Your body is resting on a bed and your head is resting on a pillow. You are likely wearing sleepwear unless you choose to sleep sans clothing. The materials in contact with your skin—your bedding, your pillowcase, and your pajamas—can have a direct impact on the quality of your sleep.

—

The Perfect Pillow

Every night you place your head on a pillow that is wrapped in a pillowcase. If you are like the majority of people, you have not given this pillow or this pillowcase much thought. Perhaps the pillows were bought in a pack of two at a department store or they were gifted to you. Perhaps the pillowcase came included with a sheet set or maybe it was included with the pillow.

It seems a little crazy that we are taught to put so much time and effort into picking out our clothing—which we change daily—but very little thought into picking out our pillow and pillowcase—which we rest our face against for about 8 hours every single night.

Pillows absorb dust, saliva, bacteria, and mold. It is important to replace your pillow regularly so that these allergens don't impact your health. If your pillow has any stains or discoloration, it's time for a new pillow.

PILLOW PARAMETERS

When picking out your perfect pillow, you have to identify your sleeping position and your support needs.

- **Side sleeper:** you likely need a pillow that's firm and thick. This thickness helps provide the support needed to cradle your neck and head. You may want to use a wool, latex, or memory foam pillow because they tend to be thicker than others.

- **Back sleeper:** you'll need a slightly flatter pillow that is comfortable and supportive. This is all about keeping your neck in alignment with your spine. Pillows made of cotton and down can provide adequate support.

- **Stomach sleeper:** you'll need a very flat pillow or no pillow at all. You can also use pillows underneath your hips or knees to help keep yourself in alignment.

There are also numerous pillow innovations on the market, such as pillows made specifically for your sleeping position and pillows that are adjustable with a variety of different sized inserts to adapt to your particular support needs. A quick internet search will provide you with a variety of options suited for you.

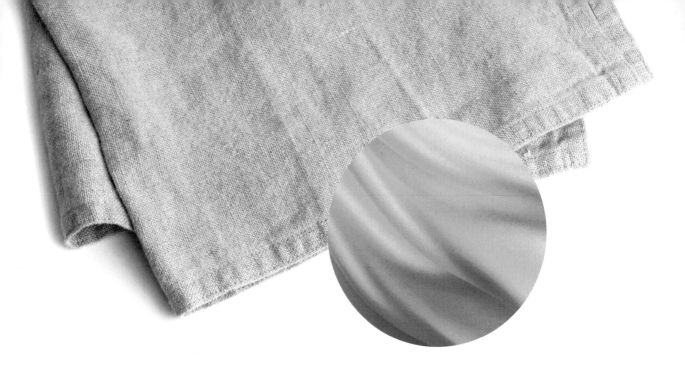

Pillowcase Fabric Options

- **Cotton:** this light and breathable fabric is easy to wash. If you are looking for a smoother feel against your skin, opt for a higher thread count. There are also a variety of sub-options within the cotton pillowcase category. One example is jersey, a 100% cotton material that feels super soft—like your favorite T-shirt that you've worn and washed more times than you can count. One of the negatives of cotton pillowcases is that they can leave creases on your face, which can lead to wrinkles.

- **Linen:** Linen is an ideal choice if you live somewhere with hot or muggy summers because it is very breathable. Some people opt to switch their pillowcase out based on the season, so linen is a good choice for your spring and summer pillowcase. Linen pillowcases can be machine-washed and they get softer each and every time you wash them.

- **Silk:** this luxurious fabric is a little pricier than other options. It's also higher-maintenance, as it's recommended that you hand wash silk pillowcases. However, the extra effort might be worth it because silk pillowcases are the best for your skin. Silk is cleaner because it does not absorb moisture, oil, or bacteria like cotton does, and its smooth surface helps reduce friction and irritation that might cause wrinkles or acne.

- **Satin:** this fabric is not as luxurious as silk, but it has a smooth feeling, is easier on the bank account, and can be machine washed. It also helps keep your hair smooth and frizz-free.

- **Copper:** this relatively new pillowcase concept touts anti-microbial benefits. It is thought to kill pillow-related bacteria that can produce acne. Additionally, as copper is necessary for collagen production and collagen is a skin superhero, this type of pillowcase may aid in wrinkle prevention and reduction.

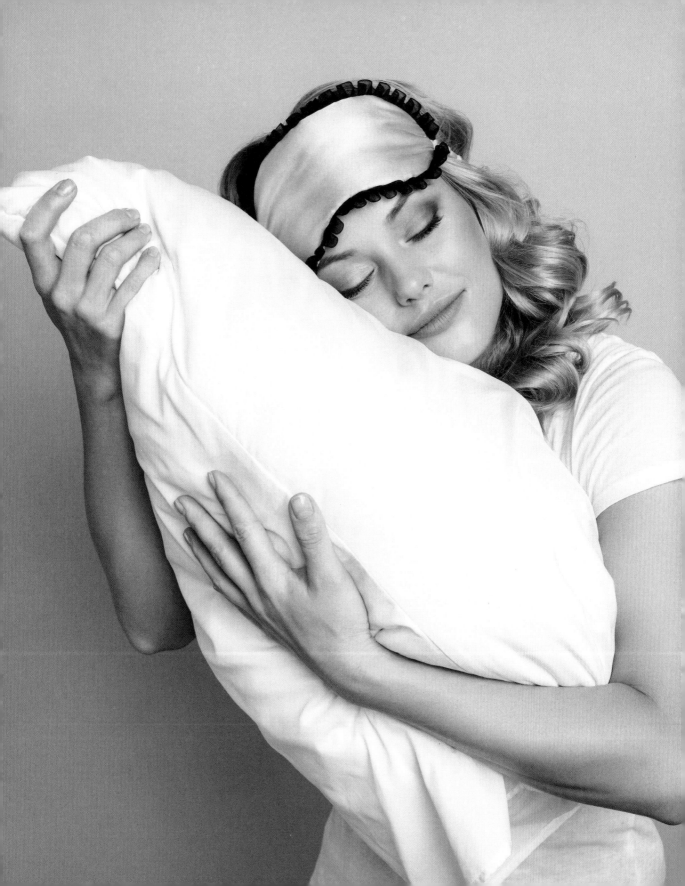

Mattress Matters

The average mattress lasts for 6–12 years. If you've owned your mattress for this amount of time or you received a hand-me-down mattress from family or friends, it's time for an upgrade.

Though mattresses are not inexpensive, they are worth the investment. You spend close to one third of your life in bed, so you ought to make it comfortable and beneficial to your health.

Ideally, it is best to try out mattresses in person. When going to the store, have your mattress needs in mind, and try out a few different mattresses that meet your parameters. Spend at least ten minutes on each mattress to adequately assess. If you have a dominant sleeping position, lie on the mattress for 10 minutes in that position. You should feel comfortable, yet solidly supported.

If you are unable to try out a mattress in person, there are many companies that sell mattresses online and offer risk-free returns. You can try out a mattress for a month (or even longer!) and return it if it doesn't fit your sleep needs.

Before purchasing a mattress, you will need to determine two things:
1. The material you prefer.
2. The firmness you require.

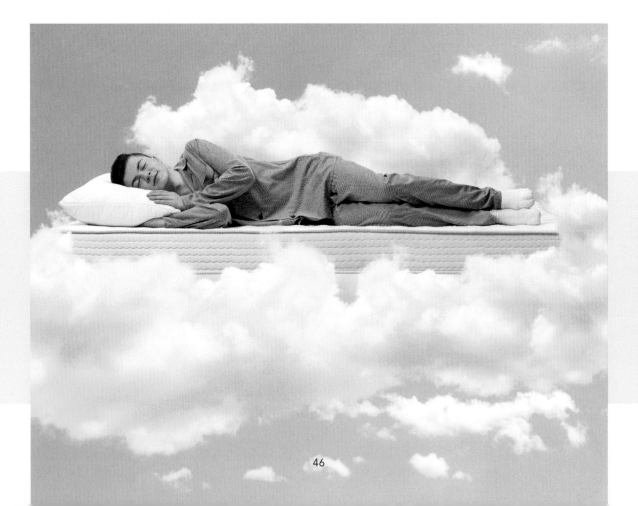

MATTRESS MATERIALS

- **Foam:** this material is a good choice for side sleepers because it contours to the body and offers pressure relief. As memory foam transfers the least amount of motion, it is a good choice for couples who share a bed. On the downside, this mattress might not be for you if you run warm while you sleep, because it can trap body heat. If you're a hot sleeper, find a memory foam mattress that incorporates cooling features.

- **Innerspring:** internal coils are the source of support in this mattress, but they are not the best choice for those, like side sleepers, who need pressure relief. This type of mattress is a good option for a stomach sleeper or for people who weigh more than 200 pounds. This mattress is also the most budget-friendly. This mattress does transfer motion, so if you are sharing the bed with someone who moves frequently throughout the evening, it may not be the best option.

- **Hybrid:** this mattress is a combination of a foam mattress and an innerspring. The foam component is placed on top of the innerspring component. This mattress is a good middle ground. It isn't as budget-conscious as the innerspring mattress, but it is typically more affordable than a memory foam mattress. It offers some support and moderate pressure relief and transfers less motion than an innerspring mattress, so couples can sleep soundly side by side. This mattress is a solid choice for stomach and back sleepers.

- **Latex:** this type of mattress is very durable and is able to efficiently contour to the body. This mattress is great if you change sleeping positions throughout the night because it is responsive and supportive. However, if you share a bed with your partner you may disturb your sleeping companion because this bouncy mattress transfers motion.

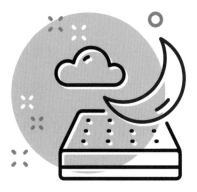

MATTRESS FIRMNESS

- **Medium soft to medium firm:** this level of firmness is best for side sleepers who need support on their shoulders and hips.

- **Medium firm to firm:** a slightly firmer mattress is best for back sleepers who need support for their lower back.

- **Firm:** this is the best option for stomach sleepers who need a source of fairly rigid support.

The two extremes in firmness—soft and extra firm—are reserved for those who fall into certain weight categories. If you are under 130 pounds, you may benefit from a soft mattress. If you are over 230 pounds and sleep on your stomach, you may benefit from an extra firm mattress.

If you are unsure as to which firmness is best for you, medium firm is a safe choice because it is the firmness that is most often used in hotels as it has the widest appeal.

Sleepy Sheets

Each night when you get in bed, you wrap yourself up in your sheets. The fabric you choose for your sheets is important. For breathability, sustainability, and ease of care, nothing beats cotton. Cotton allows air flow and can be machine washed and dried. When purchasing cotton sheets, you want to pay attention to the thread count and the weave.

When it comes to thread count, higher isn't always better. Sometimes the higher thread counts listed are a bit deceptive, and thinner thread is used to up the thread count—which means that a higher thread count may result in a higher price tag, but an inferior product. Do not get sheets with less than a 200 thread count—anything lower might be scratchy or poorly made. Also, do not waste your money on sheets over a 600 thread count. Your 600 thread count sheets will be soft against your skin and will get softer with each wash.

The weave of the cotton makes one of the biggest differences when it comes to the sheets you choose. The five common cotton weaves for sheets are as follows:

- **Flannel:** these sheets are incredibly soft and a little bit warmer than the other cotton finishes, as this material traps heat.

- **Jersey Knit:** technically this is a knit and not a weave, but it is a traditional finish for cotton sheets. This feels like a super soft worn-in T-shirt.

- **Percale:** when you think of crisp white hotel sheets, you're likely thinking of percale sheets. This is a durable fabric that will hold up to being washed. It's also a great choice for hot sleepers because it is quite light and breathable.

- **Combed Cotton:** this fabric has been "combed" to remove the short cotton fibers. This increases both the softness and strength of the fabric.

- **Sateen:** this weave makes the sheets feel satin-like. This weave will be quite soft and a bit heavier than other options. This weave helps keep you warm if you are a cold sleeper.

Note: if you are a super hot sleeper and need the lightest and most breathable option, you might be the exception to the cotton-sheet-suggestion. Try linen sheets for the absolute lightest option out there.

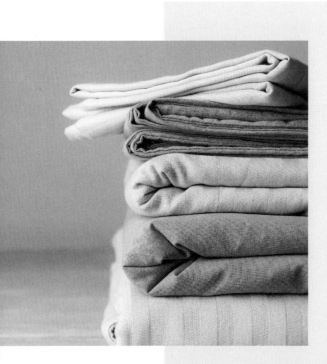

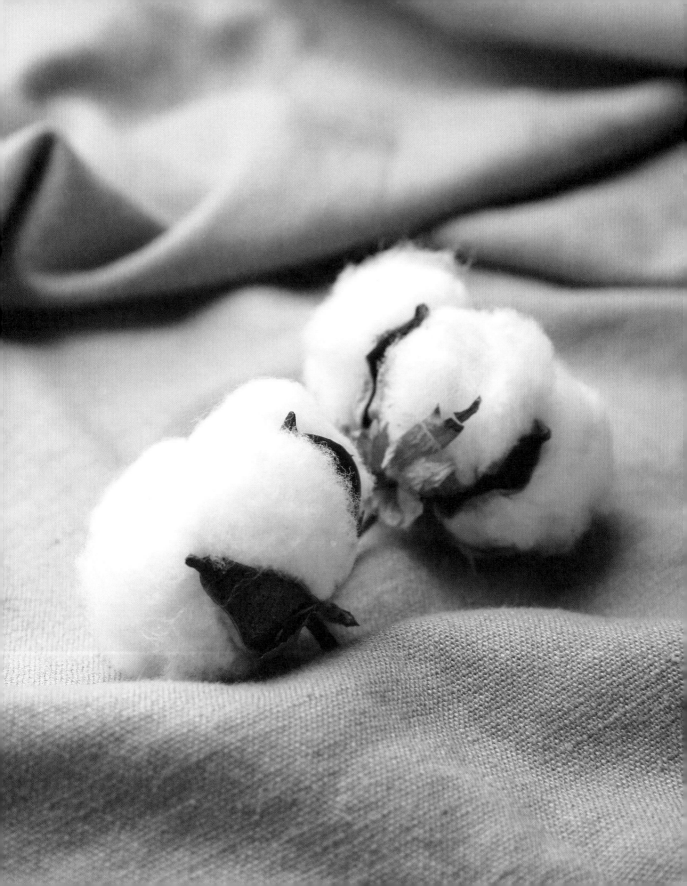

Sleepwear for Optimum Comfort

When it comes to choosing sleepwear, think about your sheets. When you find a sheet fabric that works for you, the pajamas you choose can mirror your choice. Do you feel amazing sleeping in jersey sheets? Search for a jersey sleep set. Do you absolutely love the coziness of flannel sheets? Flannel pajamas are readily available.

If you are someone who likes things to feel indulgent, luxurious, or just have a thing for smooth fabric, you may want to invest in some silk sleepwear. This is a much more affordable option than a set of expensive silk sheets and works well with cotton sheets for movement and breathability.

When it comes to sleepwear, the only thing that matters more than the fabric is the fit. Look for items that aren't too tight because this can constrict your movements while you sleep. Also, don't buy items that are too oversized. Oversized items can twist around you as you move during the night, leading to fitful sleep. A simple way to buy comfortable sleepwear is to buy items one size larger than your normal, fitted, daytime clothing.

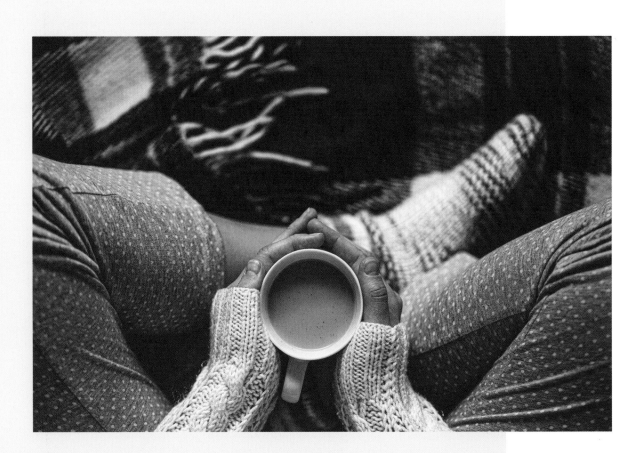

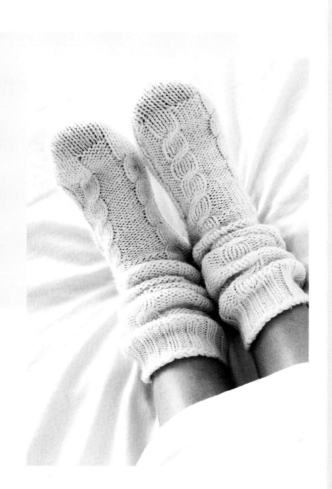

Socks – An Overlooked Sleep Aid

Socks that are cozy and fitted, but not tight, may help you fall asleep and stay asleep. When your feet warm up, the blood vessels dilate. This allows the heat to move toward the extremities of your body, which signals to the brain that it is time to go to bed. It has been shown that the greater the blood vessel dilation in the feet, the less time it takes to arrive in dreamland.

Sleepytime Fabric Analysis Exercise

Ask yourself the following questions. Any question to which your answer is "no" is an indication that you should reassess and improve this element of your bedroom.

Is your pillow comfortable and supportive?

Do you wake up without any neck and shoulder pain?

Is your pillow less than eighteen months old?

When you wake up, is your face crease-free?

Is your mattress comfortable and supportive?

Do you wake up without any joint or muscle pain in your body?

Is your mattress less than six years old?

Do you like the way your sheets feel against your skin?

Does your body temperature feel comfortable throughout the night?

Do you like your selection of sleepwear?

Does your sleepwear fit you comfortably: not too tight, not too loose?

Do you sleep in socks?

The Influence of Color

Color psychology is the understanding that different colors stimulate different emotions. The colors around us have a subconscious impact on our mood, mindset, and nervous system. When applied to the realm of interior design, you can utilize specific colors in your home to achieve a desired emotional effect.

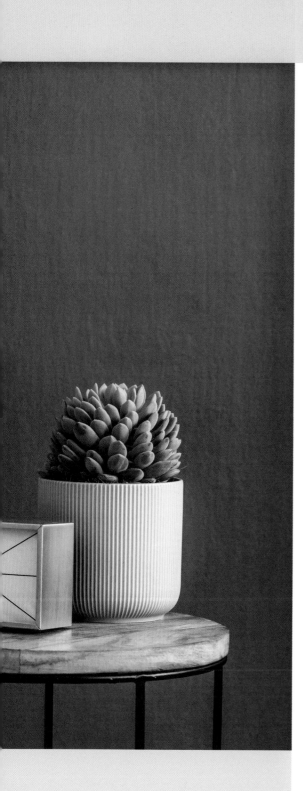

When incorporating colors into the bedroom, it is important to prioritize calming hues that signal to the body and brain that it is time to rest, relax, and unwind. The following colors have psychological benefits that are ideal for the bedroom.

———

Blue: this color lowers pulse rate and body temperature. Many people find blue to be calming, tranquil, and serene. Blue is associated with the color of the water and the sky, both relaxing natural elements.

Green: this is the color most often found in the natural world. Trees, plants, and grass are green. Green is the color associated with nature, so it invokes feelings of balance, growth, and restoration.

White: this color is associated with purity. It is also calming because it feels clean, minimal, and fresh. To ensure that white does not feel too cold, you can choose creamy white hues that have an element of warmth to them.

Brown: this is the color of the earth, dirt, and mud. This causes it to be a very grounding color. This can make you feel balanced, centered, and connected.

Pink: when this color is bright, it can be energizing. However, when pink is presented in a soft, muted, or pastel shade, it is soothing and invokes feelings of kindness, being nurtured, and a sense of calm.

Gray: this neutral shade is calming for many, but be aware of the way it impacts you as an individual. For some, this foggy hue is relaxing, like reading a book inside on a rainy day. For others, it can invoke a feeling of sadness or depression, like encountering a gray day at the beach.

Using Color to Calm

Now that you understand the basics of color psychology, you can apply this knowledge to the decor in your bedroom.

(1) **Start with a fairly neutral canvas.** First remove all bold colors from your room. These colors include red, orange, yellow, and black. These colors stimulate energy, motivation, inspiration, and aggression. These attributes can be positive, but they are not conducive to an environment for rest.

(2) **Pick one or two shades from the colors listed above.** Pick your favorite hues or look at other items you own and see if you already have some decor items that fall into a certain color category.

(3) **Gather or purchase decor items in that color.** Use these items to adorn your bedroom. Simple ways to incorporate the colors you have chosen are in the form of throw pillows, the color of your bedding, or a cozy blanket. You could also hang a picture that incorporates some of the calming colors listed above.

For example: if you chose the colors white and blue, you may want to purchase a white comforter for your bed, a couple of muted blue throw pillows, and a painting of the ocean in a white frame. If you chose the colors brown and green, you might want to paint one of your bedroom walls a sage green color and place potted plants around your room. The possibilities are as limitless as your imagination.

(4) **After you decorate your room with calming colors, assess how you feel.** Do you notice that you feel more at peace in your space? If you are looking to feel peaceful in your home, you can incorporate color psychology into other rooms. For inspiration, you can start with the bathroom that you use to prepare yourself for bed.

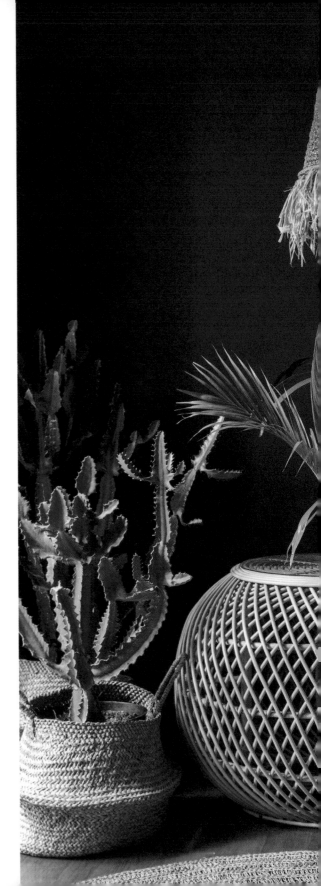

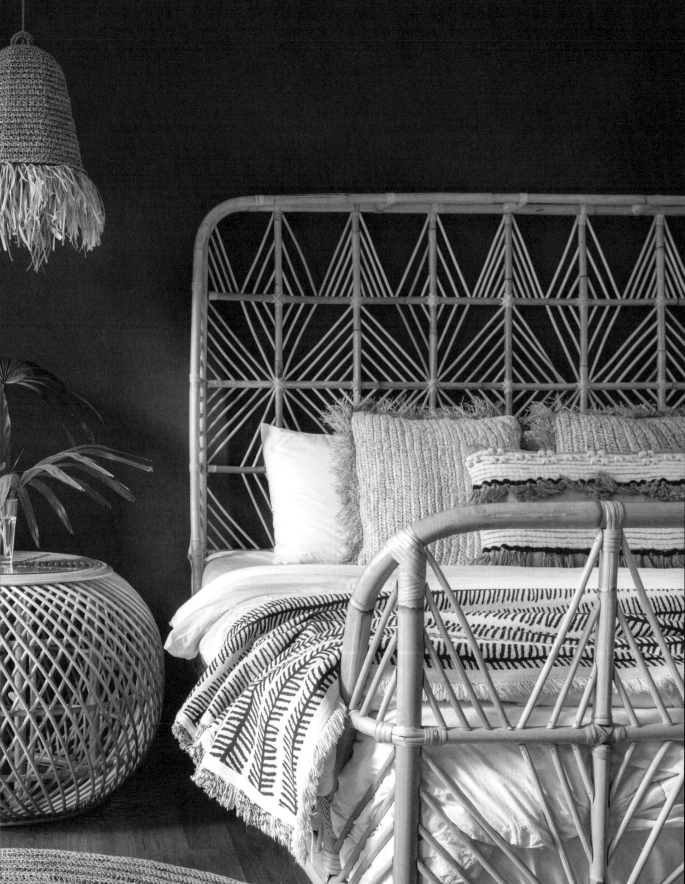

The Power of Light

As mentioned in Chapter One, your circadian rhythm is a powerful internal process that uses light to help regulate sleeping and waking patterns. If you would like your circadian rhythm to assist you with sleep, you can focus on providing it with appropriately timed soothing sources of light.

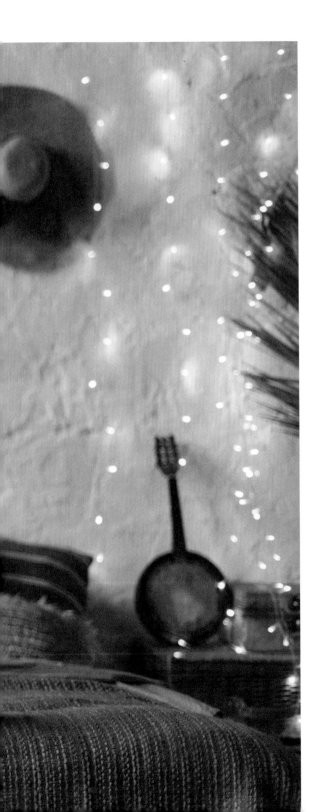

How to Layer the Lighting in Your Sanctuary

Have you ever heard of layering your lighting? It's a concept utilized by many interior designers to influence the mood of a space.

To understand what layered lighting is, let's first identify what it is not. Non-layered lighting is present in any room that receives light from a single source. Think of a dining room lit by a chandelier. It's the kind of room that you walk into, flip a light switch, and the sole source of light in the room turns on.

Now imagine a room with an overhead light, lamps placed on side tables, a floor lamp, and some cabinets with built-in lighting. This room has many sources of light that can be turned on and off to create different combinations, strengths, and sources of light. This kind of a room may even have lights that are attached to dimmers, timers, and a variety of switches.

Layered lighting in a home allows you to adjust the amount of light you are absorbing throughout the day and night. This can provide an experience more in tune with the natural light patterns of the sun. This means that layered lighting, when used correctly, can more appropriately activate your body's circadian rhythm.

For layered lighting to work optimally, you also want to have a way to control the external light that you allow into a room. If your bedroom gets a lot of sunlight or moonlight, you may want to invest in blackout shades to better control the light cues that you are sending to your brain.

Lumens vs. Watts

You may have heard of watts before. Traditionally, different light bulbs had different wattages and that is how the strength of the light was determined. Wattage was never intended to measure the brightness of a light. Watts are a measure of how much energy a lightbulb uses. Because most light bulbs used to operate the same way, the wattage used to be a reliable way to estimate the brightness of the bulb.

Now that there are a variety of types of lights—like LED vs. incandescent—the watts, are no longer a solid indication of the amount of light that the bulb emits. This is because different types of lights can produce different levels of brightness using the same amount of watts.

To determine the strength of the light, you will want to take note of the lumens. Lumens are a measure of the amount of light emitted from the bulb.

For your bedroom, you will want to aim for gentler and softer light. This falls somewhere around 800 lumens.

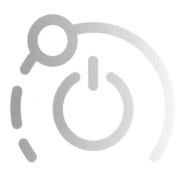

The Warmth of Your Light

You may have noticed that some artificial light bulbs emit a bright white light (think fluorescent lighting), while others emit a warm orange-toned light (think a dimly lit hotel bar). The difference in these colors is measured in Kelvins.

Kelvins literally measure temperature. It is this temperature difference that is responsible for the different shades of light. The higher the Kelvins, the whiter, colder, and brighter the light. The lower the Kelvins, the yellower, warmer, and cozier the light.

For your bedroom, the ideal range falls somewhere around 2700 and 3000 Kelvins. Oftentimes, bulbs in this range will read "soft white" light.

Dimmers and Timers

Your lighting may be hardwired to a dimming switch already. If it's not, you can go the DIY route and install your own dimmer switches. If you are handy, this should be fairly easy for you. If you are not handy—no judgment here!—there are some new advancements in technology that allow you to have dimmable lights without a dimmer switch. The main benefit of dimmable lights is that you control how much light your eyes are exposed to at any given time. It also helps you control the mood in an environment.

Another helpful addition is syncing your lights to timers. One way to do this is to install smart outlets. Smart outlets allow you to control the outlet without having to turn on and off a physical switch With these outlets, you can use your phone or your voice to control your lights. You can set them to turn on and off at set times or on command. You can even set a timer.

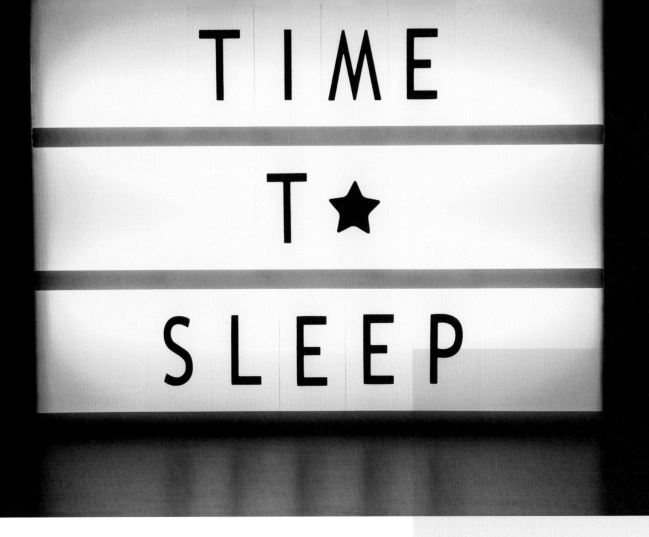

If you do not have or do not want to install a dimmer or smart outlets, you have another option. Today's smart bulbs only need to be screwed into a light source and synced to your phone. Though this option is a bit more expensive, it offers ease of installation and a lot of different options to control your lighting experience. These light bulbs allow you to dim the light, sync them to timers, and even change the color and hue of the bulb.

Banishing Blue Light

Blue light is the light that is emitted from screens and many energy-efficient LED bulbs. The lighting in your house, your television screen, tablet, computer, and phone are all sources of blue light. During the day, blue light can be helpful because it has been found to keep people alert, but it is highly disruptive at night. Blue light is the most disruptive of all colors of light to the secretion of melatonin, which is a hormone that helps you sleep.

You can minimize blue light using the following simple steps:

- Make your bedroom a screen-free environment. No television screens, laptops, tablets, or phones. Instead of using your phone as your morning alarm, invest in an alarm clock.

- If you can't part with your phone while you sleep, move it across the room. Additionally, do not look at it for a couple of hours before bed. You can also warm up the light on your phone by changing your phone settings or place it in Night Mode.

- Utilize blue light blocking glasses in the evening.

- Make sure that all lightbulbs in your bedroom emit soft, cozy, and warm light.

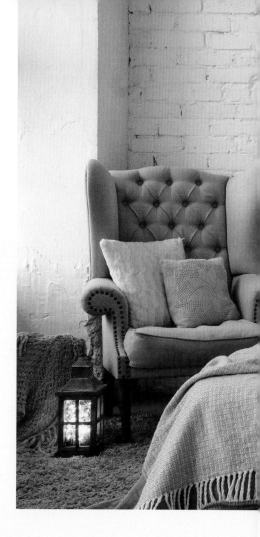

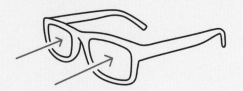

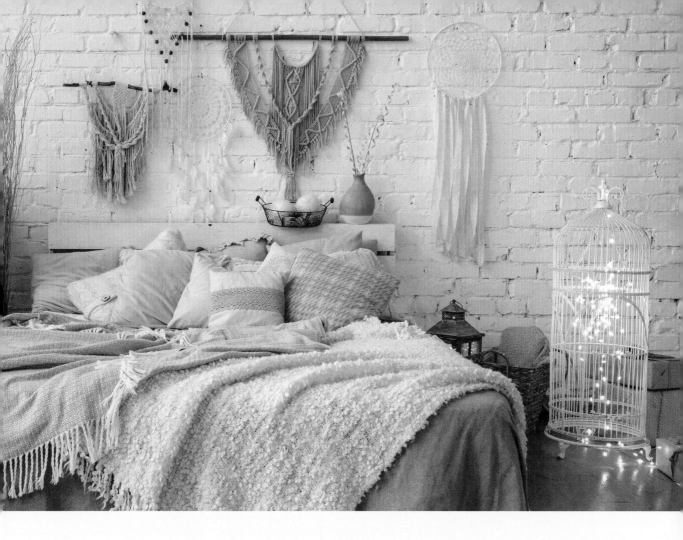

Light It Up

To benefit from the concepts above, do a quick light assessment of your bedroom.

If you have a single source of bedroom lighting, think about incorporating bedside lamps and/or a floor lamp.

When you look at your lightbulbs, consider making the switch to soft-white, energy-efficient bulbs that have the built-in ability to be placed on a dimmer, timer, or both. If you have an attached bathroom or closet that produces light, you should assess this lighting, as well. Replace these bulbs if needed.

If you do not have the finances to switch out bulbs, you can soften light from a lamp by throwing a sheer scarf over the shade. Do not leave this unattended, as it can be a fire hazard.

Once you have all of this in place, sync your lights to your circadian rhythm. This can be done by looking up the time for sunset and setting all of the lights in the bedroom to begin to dim at that point. Alternatively, you can set an alarm on your phone to remind you to dim the lights manually. If you are using an app or timed program, you can schedule the bulbs to get slightly dimmer each hour after sunset so that your circadian rhythm does not get disturbed.

While you sleep, you breathe deeply. As sleep assists with the removal of toxins from your brain and body, the last thing you want to do is to be inhaling toxins while you rest. Additionally, the humidity and temperature of the air around you can either interrupt your sleep or facilitate deeper sleep.

The Perfect Houseplants for Healthy Sleep

Houseplants are a wonderful addition to your sleep sanctuary. Not only are they beautiful and found to be relaxing, but they can assist with eliminating toxins in the air and create a more oxygen-rich environment.

Three low-maintenance houseplants that you can incorporate into your bedroom are:

Snake plant: this bold and spiky plant is a first time houseplant owner's dream. It tolerates all kinds of light and only needs water every 2–8 weeks. Touch the top of the soil to figure out the right watering time. If it's moist, check back next week. If it's dry, it's time to water.

Monstera plant: this lush, tropical plant with large glossy leaves is dramatic, beautiful, and easygoing. Monsteras need water about once a week. Once the soil is 50% dry to the touch, you can add more water. This plant needs sufficient drainage and doesn't like harsh sunlight.

Pothos: this plant with endless vines is perfect for a houseplant beginner. The pothos does not need a lot of care and attention just occasional watering. Stick your finger in the soil and if the top inch is dry, it's time to water. If not, check back in a couple of days.

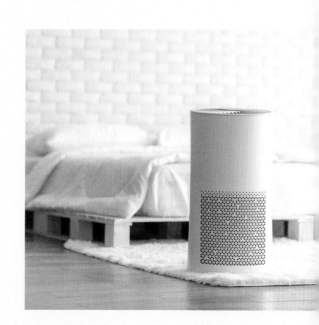

Do You Need an Air Purifier?

An air purifier is slightly different from an air filter. An air filter does exactly what it sounds like—it filters the air. Air filters remove particles from the air that are larger than the passthrough area of the internal filter. An air purifier actually purifies the air. It does this by sanitizing the particles.

To get the most efficient system, opt for an air purifier with an internal filtration system. This allows the filter to remove larger particles and sanitize some of the particles that might make it through the filter. This system can help decrease allergens, toxins, and mold.

If you are prone to allergies or are an asthma sufferer, an air purifier with a filtration system might decrease your symptoms or help eliminate them altogether. Even if you aren't prone to allergies or asthma, breathing the cleanest air possible while you sleep allows your body to work more efficiently by eliminating toxins already present in your system instead of having to battle new ones that you inhaled.

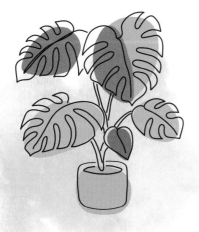

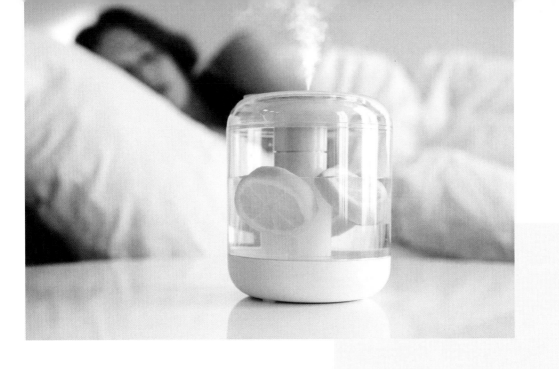

Identifying Your Ideal Temperature and Humidity

The temperature of your room can impact your ability to sleep. When it is time for rest, your internal body temperature begins to decrease. A room that is too warm will send a conflicting signal to our body, as cooler temperatures indicate that it is time to sleep. On the contrary, a room that is too cold can disrupt sleep when you have an involuntary shiver response or need to grab extra blankets in the middle of the night.

For most people, the ideal sleep temperature falls somewhere between 60 and 67 degrees. Try setting your thermostat within this range and then adjust it a degree or two each week to find your favorite temperature. If you do not have a space in which you can easily control the temperature, you may want to invest in a space heater or a portable air conditioning unit.

In addition to the temperature of the air around you, the humidity, or the amount of water vapor in the air, can impact your ability to sleep. If the humidity is too high, it can trigger everything from allergies to sweating. If this makes it difficult for you to sleep, you will not cycle all the way into the most restorative deep sleep stages.

Humidity is a personal choice, but should fall somewhere within the range of 30%-60%. If you wake up with dry skin or a parched throat, you may need to increase the humidity in your room. Other benefits to increasing the humidity in your room include plumper skin and fewer wrinkles.

You can increase the humidity in your room by purchasing a humidifier. You can purchase a bedside humidifier that works only to increase the humidity in your immediate sleeping vicinity. These humidifiers are oftentimes small, affordable, portable, and even stylish.

Prioritizing the Air Around You Exercise

Take a moment to assess your sleeping environment and make any necessary changes to your sanctuary to improve your air quality and overall sleep experience.

① Before you go to sleep, get into bed. Take note of the temperature. Is it comfortable? Look around your room. Do you have any houseplants? Breathe deeply. Do you feel like the air in your room is as pure as it could be?

② When you wake up, ask yourself the following questions before getting out of bed. Take note of the temperature. Is it comfortable? Swallow. Does your throat feel parched? Touch the skin on your face. Does it feel like it could benefit from hydration or moisturizer?

③ If the temperature isn't too your liking, try one of the following:

• Change the setting on your thermostat

• Purchase a space heater

• Purchase an air conditioning unit

• Buy a fan

④ If you don't have any houseplants, go and get one! You can use the suggested plants in this section as a starting point or purchase any plant that you find to be beautiful.

⑤ It never hurts to filter the air that you breathe. Check out different air filtration systems that are available. There are systems that filter the air in a single room, air throughout the home, and even built-in ones you can connect to your HVAC unit.

⑥ If the humidity in your room could use a little boost, invest in a personal humidifier. If you share the room with a partner, you may want to purchase a larger humidifier that can control the humidity in the entire room and not just at your bedside.

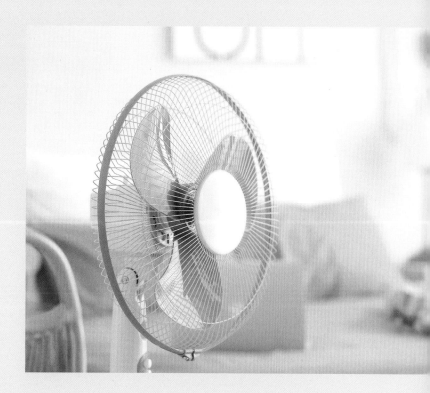

Scents for Sleep

Essential oils are scented concentrates that are created from herbs and plants. These oils have many uses, but one of the most powerful ways to use the oils is to positively impact your state of mind. Essential oils can stimulate the limbic system in your brain. This is the system that is connected to emotions, memory, blood pressure, breathing, and heart rate.

Essential oils can calm anxiety, help you feel centered, and even signal to your body that it is time for rest. You can use some oils topically. You can also diffuse them or sprinkle them onto your pillow for a full sleep sensory experience.

—

Essential Oils – The Three You Need

There are countless essential oils and essential oil blends available. If you are seeking essential oils that aid your sleep journey, the following three oils are easy to find and form a solid foundation for a relaxing aromatherapy practice.

Lavender: this floral essential oil has a soothing, earthy scent. Try sprinkling some on your pillowcase to reap the benefits while you sleep.

- Decreases anxiety
- Promotes relaxation
- Battles insomnia
- Lifts depression
- Fights allergies

Chamomile: this oil is made from the flowers of daisies. Try putting this oil in a diffuser to breathe in the chamomile-scented air deeply to prepare your body for sleep.

- Promotes sleep
- Relieves anxiety
- Anti-inflammatory benefits

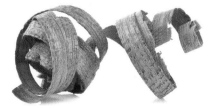

Cedarwood: much like the name implies, this oil smells like the bark of a cedar tree. This is a very earthy and grounding scent. Try adding a few drops to lotion to give yourself a calming foot massage before bed.

- •Aids in emotional balance
- Enhances relaxation
- Promotes a sense of calm
- Make Your Own Scented Lotion
- For the simplest essential oil scented lotion, you only need the following:
- Your favorite unscented body lotion
- Your favorite calming essential oil

Take some of your lotion and put it in your hand. Add a few drops of your favorite skin-safe essential oil. Rub your hands together to incorporate the oil and the lotion. Give yourself a soothing foot massage to signal to your body and brain that it is time for sleep.

Using a Diffuser – Mist or Reed

If you wanted a humidifier in the earlier section, you may want a mist diffuser. These diffusers release water particles into the air to disperse the essential oil, which has the added benefit of increasing the air's humidity.

If you are looking for a simple, affordable, and aesthetically pleasing way to scent your space, try a reed diffuser. These diffusers let off a very subtle scent that lightly fills the space. You can create your own reed diffuser with a small glass jar and a few bamboo skewers. Take 20–30 drops of your essential oil and add it to ¼ cup of fractionated coconut oil and a tablespoon of rubbing alcohol. Mix together and add to your glass jar. Stick your bamboo skewers in the jar and allow them to soak up the mixture overnight. In the morning, flip the skewers over. Replace the oil blend and skewers in the bottle after a month or two

Sleep Sounds to Soothe

Sound is a very powerful and oftentimes overlooked modality that can impact sleep. The frequency of sound can impact the frequency of your brainwaves. As your brainwaves shift with each phase of sleep, you can utilize sound frequencies to make the sleep experience more efficient. Simply stated: the right sounds can help relax your mind.

You can intentionally incorporate sound into your sleep sanctuary to further enhance your sleep environment.

—

Mastering Sound Frequencies

The various stages of sleep are outlined in detail in Chapter One. This section explains each type of brain wave or frequency that is associated with each stage of sleep.

The First Stage of Sleep - Falling Asleep
The initial stage of sleep is associated with two types of brain waves: alpha and theta. Alpha waves are fairly low frequency waves associated with a range of 8–13 Hz. In this state you are awake, but relaxed. Theta waves are even lower frequency waves associated with a range of 4–7 Hz.

The Second Stage of Sleep - Light Sleep
During the second stage of sleep, theta waves take over. Though theta waves dominate this sleep phase, they are occasionally interrupted by sleep spindles - bursts of higher frequency brain waves.

The Third Stage of Sleep - Deep Sleep
When you transition to deep sleep, the most restorative and regenerative phase of sleep, your brain waves shift to an even lower frequency. This lower frequency wave is called a delta wave which is associated with a frequency of up to 4 Hz.

The Fourth Stage of Sleep - Dream Sleep
While you are in REM sleep, your brain waves appear to be quite similar to your brain waves when you are awake.

To initiate sleep—and to stay asleep—your brain needs to downshift into the slower, or lower frequency, brainwaves. You can assist this process by incorporating lower frequency theta and delta waves into your space.

Identify Your Favorite Binaural Beats

Imagine you are hearing one sound in your left ear and another sound in your right ear. Your brain processes each sound frequency separately and registers the difference between the two. Your brain would create the auditory illusion of hearing a third frequency —the frequency difference between the sound in your left ear and the sound in your right ear. This third frequency is known as a binaural beat.

Binaural beats are effective at promoting relaxation, entering a meditative state, decreasing anxiety, diminishing stress and facilitating sleep.

To put this into practice, you want to identify the frequency you are trying to achieve. As we know that theta waves and delta waves are the most helpful to achieve deep sleep, you will want to aim for one of these frequencies. Based on this information, you will want to choose a frequency under 7 Hz.

You can do a quick internet search for "binaural beats for sleep" or you can create your own binaural beats using tools online and smartphone apps. You can also look up music that utilizes binaural beats as part of the composition.

Once you have your preferred method of listening to binaural beats, lie down and close your eyes. Using headphones, listen to the beats for at least thirty minutes to achieve the desired effect.

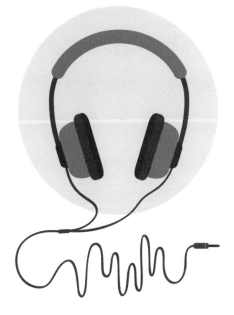

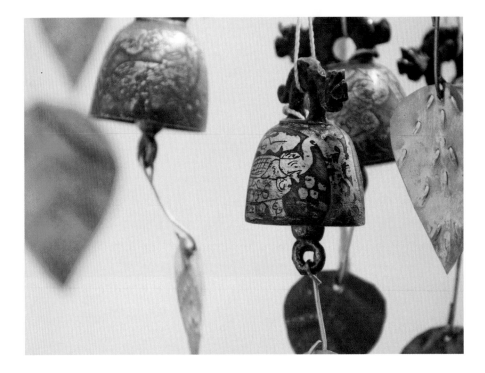

Take a Sound Bath at Home

The name "sound bath" is a literal description of the experience: you are bathed in sound. A traditional sound bath involves lying down and allowing a practitioner to play a series of sounds —some created with the human voice, some with instruments tuned to a specific frequency, and others that incorporate rhythms or natural sounds—to enter a meditative state. You may experience chanting, vibration, the beat of a drum, or the sounds of a rainstick. Each sound bath is unique. The practice of being healed by sound has been around for thousands of years.

Sound baths can be used to enter a state of relaxation and lessen anxiety. Due to this, incorporating a sound bath to assist with falling asleep could be beneficial to you.

You do not always need a practitioner to experience the benefits of a sound bath. The internet and music servers have countless resources to experience a sound bath within the comfort of your own home. You can explore a variety of sound bath tracks available online until you find one that works for you.

An important element of a sound bath is being surrounded by the sound. You should feel like it is enveloping you, almost like you are floating in a sea of sound. To achieve this, you can utilize headphones or a set of speakers on either side of you. Lie down, close your eyes, hit play, and listen. Breathe deeply during the experience and allow yourself to be transported— or just allow yourself to fall asleep!

SINGING BOWLS

Many sound baths use bowls that are tuned to a specific frequency. These bowls are commonly referred to as singing bowls or sound bowls. They come in a variety of materials, are quite beautiful, and make a lovely addition to any bedroom. You can find singing bowls made of metal and crystal with crystal having more consistent, clearer sound.

To pick a sound bowl for sleep, you want one that is tuned around 432 Hz. This frequency is associated with increased states of relaxation and decreased states of tension. However, most singing bowls produce increased relaxation regardless of the frequency, so you can also choose a bowl based on which sound is most in tune with your personal taste.

A sound bowl is "played" by running a wooden stick, known as a puja, or a leather or cloth wrapped mallet around its edge. It can also be played by using your fingers or hand. To understand the way a singing bowl works, imagine someone running their finger around the edge of a wine glass. The friction of touching the object creates a vibration along the material's edge which results in a frequency that we can hear.

You can experience singing bowls live or hire a practitioner. If, however, you would like to experience it in the comfort of your bedroom, you can utilize an internet search or even learn to play the singing bowls yourself.

You can look up "singing bowls," "sound bowls," or "singing bowls for sleep" to jump start your search. Use headphones or surround sound speakers because the same concept that applies to sound baths applies to singing bowls. Lie down and allow the sound to surround you.

If you like this practice, you can purchase your own singing bowl, multiple singing bowls, or a complete set of all the different singing bowl notes. Many people find the practice of playing the bowls to be relaxing. You can keep the bowls on display in your bedroom to further engrain this bedtime ritual in your mind.

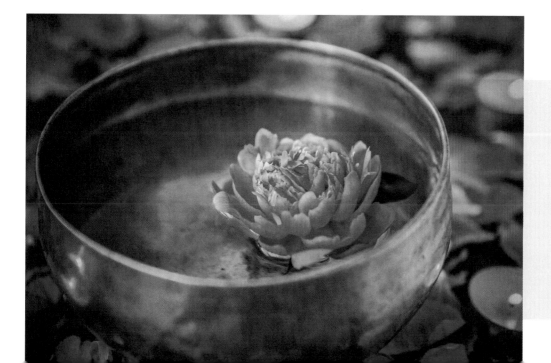

Create Your Own Soundscape

The idea of a soundscape is like a sound bath, but it utilizes modern technology. Soundscapes often incorporate pre-recorded or artificially created nature sounds in conjunction with other layered sounds, background noises, music, frequencies, or beats.

If you are someone who likes nature sounds or the sound of traditional music more than the ancient and unfamiliar sound of singing bowls, then soundscapes might be for you.

There are many smartphone apps available that allow you to listen to a previously created soundscape or even create your own. To create your own soundscape, download a smartphone app that allows you to layer sounds. These apps come with a series of pre-recorded sounds, music, and even binaural beats. Continue to layer sounds and remove sounds until you create a soundscape you enjoy.

You can also change the volume of each layered sound to make certain sounds more or less pronounced. On a personal note, I found (after much trial and error!) that I prefer the sound of a campfire to be a dominant sound layered over less dominant white noise layered over an almost inaudible low hertz frequency. Give yourself plenty of time—and multiple weeks of experimentation—before identifying your ideal soundscape.

If smartphone apps are not for you, you can purchase a sound or white noise machine. These machines come with pre-recorded sounds of nature and/or white noise. Some of them allow you to layer the sounds.

If you do not enjoy technology, incorporate a small water feature in your bedroom to enjoy the natural soundscape produced by running water.

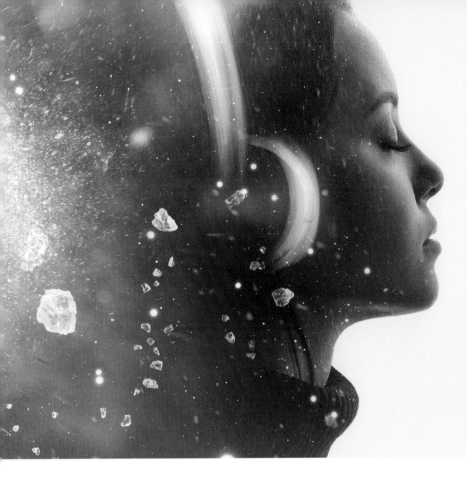

Creating Your Sleep Sanctuary Shopping List

Only partake in this exercise after you have read each section in this chapter. Once you have completed this chapter, revisit the exercise at the beginning of this chapter "Dream Your Sanctuary of Slumber." Complete the exercise for a second time. This time, use the list you created the first time around as a jumping off point. Add every single item you visualized in your perfect bedroom. This is your Sleep Sanctuary Shopping List.

This does not mean that you have to go and purchase all of these items right away. Identify the cost and the benefit of each item. For example, a new mattress is quite expensive, but it may have a huge benefit to your sleep patterns if your current mattress doesn't make the cut. On the other hand, houseplants aren't very expensive—you might be able to afford one today—but they can have a wonderful impact on oxygen, enhance your sense of calm, and beautify your space.

After assessing each item on the list, re-write your list on another sheet of paper in order of priority. Make it your goal to purchase each item on this list by year's end. Think about it: twelve months from today you could go to sleep every single night in the bedroom of your dreams. As you spend about 33% of your life in your bedroom, it only takes one year to vastly improve one-third of your life.

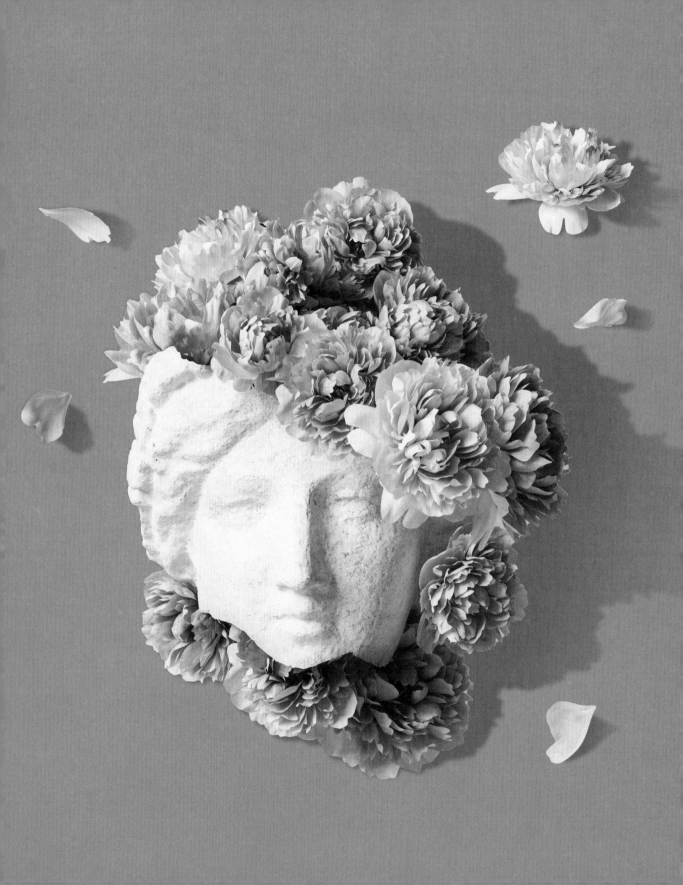

GREAT SLEEP STARTS WITHIN

Self-Care Strategies That Align Your Mind with Sand Land

*"Throw off your worries
when you throw off your
clothes at night."*

- NAPOLEON BONAPARTE -

Inner Peace = Better Sleep

The previous chapter is about curating a peaceful external environment. It addresses the importance of minimizing unnecessary stimuli and incorporating elements that promote rest. It teaches you to be aware of what helps you fall asleep and what interferes with sleep. This chapter is going to be similar, but you will be assessing the *environment within yourself*.

In a perfect world, you would be able to fall asleep on command. You would lie down, close your eyes, fall asleep immediately, and sleep for eight hours to wake rested and refreshed.

———

In the real world, things are different. You can make the decision to go to bed when you like, but that does not necessarily equate with falling asleep. Your night might look like this: you lie down and close your eyes. Suddenly, you remember you have a presentation at work next week. Your mind becomes fixated on this and sends waves of stress through your body. You try to calm down, but it takes another hour for you to fall asleep. Ninety minutes later you wake up and need to use the restroom. After using the restroom, you stumble back to bed and lie down. You are wide awake, but tired. You stare at the ceiling for thirty minutes until you fall back asleep. You wake up three hours later. You check the time and realize your alarm is going to go off in an hour. You begin to think about everything you have to do after your alarm goes off. You lie in bed with your eyes closed trying to pretend that you are getting some rest. Then your alarm goes off. You get out of bed feeling groggy, disoriented, and a little grumpy.

Our bodies and our brains do not always cooperate with our desires. You think, *"Time to sleep"* and your brain thinks, *"Time to create a mental to-do list of everything I have to do and everything I have not yet done in my life."* You think, *"Time to allow my body to relax because I've been on my feet all day"* and your body thinks, *"Time to get chilly feet, a charley horse in*

the left calf, and an overwhelming urge to drink water." This is like being at war with yourself. You can learn to incorporate new knowledge and habits that end this war once and for all.

Once you learn to work in harmony with your mind and body, you will be able to fall asleep faster and sleep more soundly. Sleep will no longer be a struggle for you. You will not feel anxious about your sleep struggles; instead, you will be able to get into bed with the feeling of peace that comes with knowing that you are going to wake well-rested in the morning.

This chapter will help you get into mind-body alignment and will provide you with easy-to-implement strategies and practices that can benefit you from the very first day.

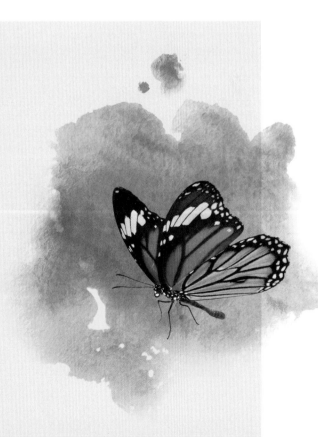

Exercise Yourself to Sleep

Physics may not have been your favorite subject in school, but it came with an important lesson. Do you remember Sir Isaac Newton's first law of motion? It states that "An object at rest stays at rest, and an object in motion stays in motion." To think about this simply: you are an object. When you are sedentary—stuck on a couch, at a desk, or sitting all day—it is customary to stay sedentary or to be an object at rest *staying at rest*. If you are active—mobile, exercising often, or walking from place to place—it is customary to stay active or to be an object in motion staying in motion.

To understand the importance of being an object in motion, think about water. When water is still and remains in one place, it becomes stagnant. Water without motion becomes a swamp. That water becomes undrinkable because it turns toxic. Now imagine running water. It might be a river, stream, or creek. Think of how clear and clean this water can be. Water in motion can is fresh and pure. The difference between toxic swamp water and fresh drinkable water is movement.

––––

Incorporating movement is also strongly recommended by health professionals. The amount of recommended exercise differs based on age. Teenagers benefit the most from daily physical activity. It is suggested that teens get sixty minutes of moderate-intensity activity each day and three days a week of vigorous-intensity and strengthening activity. Adults benefit from 150 minutes of moderate-intensity activity each week. If you prefer vigorous-intensity activity, you can satisfy your exercise recommendation by completing seventy-five minutes each week.

Once you prioritize your physical health, these recommendations are quite easy to fit into your daily life. For example, if you are an adult who enjoys moderate-intensity activity, you can satisfy your 150 minutes of weekly activity by walking thirty minutes each weekday. You can schedule this walk at the beginning of your day or fit it in after lunch to clear your head. You can even walk with a friend in the evenings to exercise while you socialize.

If you need motivation, focus on the benefits. Daily movement has both physical and mental benefits—and, yes, better sleep (falling asleep faster and sleeping longer and more deeply!) is one of the major perks. Here are just a few of the incredible benefits of getting up and getting moving:

PHYSICAL BENEFITS

- Controls weight
- Strengthens your muscles and bones
- Makes your heart healthier
- Gives you more energy
- Regulates blood sugar levels
- Increases your lifespan
- Produces antioxidants for anti-aging skin benefits
- Reduces pain
- Enhances sexual health

MENTAL BENEFITS

- Decreases anxiety and stress
- Reduces depression by increasing the sensitivity to serotonin and norepinephrine
- Increases focus and mental alertness
- Helps with memory
- Improves your mood by releasing endorphins
- Reduces stress

To ensure that you receive the sleep benefits that exercise can deliver, keep an eye on the timing of your exercise activities. As exercise causes endorphins to be released into your brain, which can give you a surge of euphoria and energy, you should finish exercising at least 2 hours before bed to give your body time to calm down. Exercise also raises your core body temperature. When you sleep, your core body temperature gets lower. The two hour window will allow your body enough time to cool down and prepare for rest.

Sweat it Out – Great Workouts for A Restful Night

The type of exercise that you choose to do is irrelevant, as any type of physical activity will produce the aforementioned benefits. It's most important to identify an activity you enjoy because you are more likely to commit to it. For many people, this means incorporating a social aspect into their exercise routine. You can join an adult sports league, take classes at a local gym, or go on hikes with your friends.

The following suggestions are great places to start. They are free, can be done with little or no exercise experience, and can be done solo or with a friend or group. Feel free to incorporate these suggestions into your weekly activity or find another way to get moving that you absolutely love.

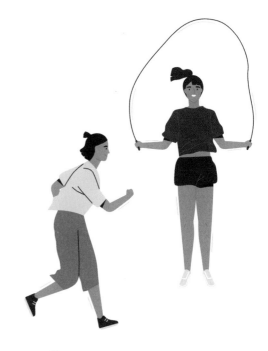

Get Walking

Walking is the easiest way to add activity to your day. All it takes is a pair of comfortable shoes. If you have a relatively sedentary lifestyle, walking is the best way to get moving. As with any physical activity, it is important that you listen to your body and not overexert yourself. The best way to achieve this is to focus on time instead of distance or pace. Start by walking slowly for thirty minutes. If you begin to fatigue during this time, do not stop; instead, slow down further. With time, you will be able to walk faster and farther.

You can choose to walk on a treadmill, but there are added benefits if you get outside. The natural light outdoors will assist your circadian rhythm (discussed at length in Chapters One and Two of this book) in syncing with the sun. You will also absorb Vitamin D, which boosts your mood and your immune system.

Once you feel capable of walking comfortably for thirty minutes, attempt these two walking challenges.

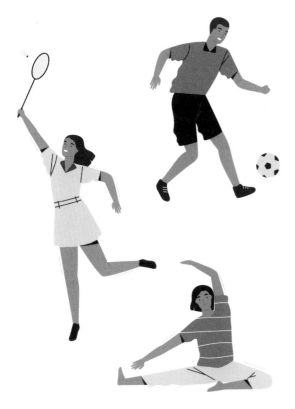

Walking Challenge #1: The Beginner

Choose a week and commit to walking for thirty minutes a day Monday through Friday. Set an alarm or a reminder to hold yourself accountable. To increase your accountability, tell a friend or co-worker about what you are doing. Sharing your goal with other people increases your accountability.

Before going on a walk, write down three words that describe how you are feeling. When you return from your walk, write down three words that describe how you are feeling. Do this each day for the five consecutive days.

Do you notice any patterns? You may find that the words you wrote upon your return were more positive than the words you wrote before going on your walk. You may also find that the words you write before going on your walk are a bit more positive each day. This is because regular exercise has residual benefits that carry over, so the boost in your mood from your walk yesterday may carry over to today.

Walking Challenge #2: 10,000 Steps

Once you complete the beginner's challenge, you may find that you begin to crave your daily walk. If you are happy with the benefits you are receiving, keep repeating the beginner's challenge. You can do this each and every week and continue to see benefits.

If, however, you feel like your fitness level can be pushed even further—which can help you achieve even deeper sleep!—you might want to dedicate more time and effort to your walking practice. Instead of thirty minutes a day, this challenge takes anywhere from an hour-and-fifteen minutes to two hours a day.

If you are thinking, *"Who has time for that? I have obligations and responsibilities,"* then utilize this time for other things, as well.

If you have phone calls to make, you can make them on your walk. If you have a book to finish, you can listen to the book on tape. If you prioritize your mental clarity, listen to meditation music. If you want to learn a new topic, find a class or podcast on it and listen while you walk. If you have emails to respond to, you can have your phone read the messages and you can dictate your responses while you move (safely, while paying attention to traffic!).

This challenge calls you to commit to walking ten thousand steps a day for thirty days. That may sound intimidating, but it is far less daunting when it's broken down. Approach each day as it comes and complete only the steps needed for that day. Ten thousand steps is approximately five miles. That's likely more than you are used to walking in a day, but it is not necessary to be in top shape to achieve this goal. It takes anywhere from 12–20 minutes to walk a mile. This means that it will take an hour to an hour and forty minutes to complete your daily steps.

Choose a month and commit to walking ten thousand steps each day of the month. Hold yourself accountable the same way that you did for the beginner's walking exercise: set an alarm or reminder, and share the fact that you are committing to this challenge with someone. Also, repeat the habit of writing three words that describe how you feel before and after the walk.

At the end of the thirty days, read all of the words that you wrote after your walk. Write all of these words down somewhere. Whenever you feel unmotivated to move, read the words you've written down as a reminder of all of the ways that movement benefits you.

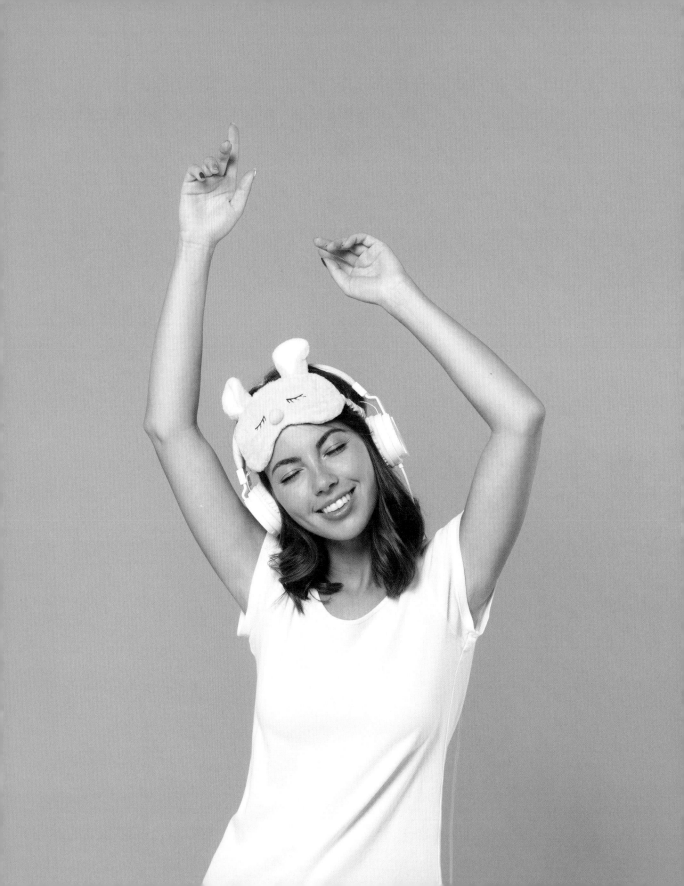

Dance It Out

Dancing is a wonderful way to get moving. When you dance, you help your body get the movement it craves, and you receive the added benefit of a major boost to your mood.

You do not need to be "good" at dancing to enjoy it. The key to enjoying dance is to give yourself permission to let loose. You might be a talented dancer—if so, feel free to dance in front of a mirror to practice your best moves. If you feel self-conscious about your dance abilities, find a private space to go at it and avoid mirrors. You have now created a safe and judgment-free zone. You can be a flailing unrhythmic whirling dervish of a dancer and still finish with a big grin on your face.

It's simple to introduce the practice of dance. You can dance freely to your favorite music at home. You can stream online dance classes. You can go to a Zumba class. You can join a ballroom dancing class. You can go to the beach, the park, or your backyard and shake it. Find a mode of dance that works for you.

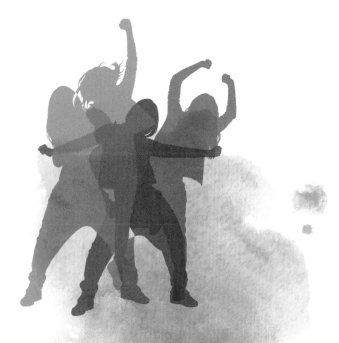

Dance at Home Exercise

① Create a thirty minute playlist of music you absolutely love. Think upbeat, inspirational, motivating, and happy. Any song that makes you want to get up and dance deserves a spot on this playlist!

② Choose a day for the exercise. By the end of the day, you will have danced to all thirty minutes of your playlist.

③ Dance for 10 minutes at the start of your day. During the first part of your day - sometime before 11am - set aside 10 minutes to dance. Set a ten-minute timer. Hit play on your playlist. Move. Dance. Jump. Crouch. Spin. *There are no rules to how* you move. Let your body move freely. Let yourself smile.

④ Dance for ten minutes twice more. Once between 11 a.m. and 3 p.m. and once between 3 p.m. and 6 p.m. repeat step three. By the end of the day you will have danced for thirty minutes.

⑤ Check in with yourself before bedtime. Did you experience more joy today than usual because of dance? If the answer is yes, this is a great indication that dance should be incorporated into your weekly exercise routine.

Eating & Drinking for Sleep

The things that you consume throughout the day—and especially close to bedtime hours—have an impact on more than just your overall health. The food you choose to eat and the beverages you choose to drink are tied directly to your sleep health.

When selecting foods and beverages for sleep, it is important to know that consuming certain things can help or hurt sleep.

—

First, the timing of when you eat your meals is important. If you eat your final meal of the day too close to bedtime, you can experience indigestion, sleep that is interrupted by the digestive process, or even acid reflux. A high-fat or spicy meal further increases the risk that your sleep will be interrupted by the digestion process. If you love high-fat, rich, or spicy foods, finish eating these kinds of foods at least four hours before you sleep. Also, avoid sweets towards the end of the day because these can stimulate your system and signal your body to stay awake.

If you are looking to enhance your sleep, there are plenty of delicious foods available that have natural properties that assist. The most important thing to notice is what vitamins, minerals, or qualities the foods possess because it is this component that aids sleep. Foods with natural melatonin, a hormone released by the brain that facilitates sleep, can aid with rest. Tryptophan is vital to the production of melatonin and serotonin, another hormone that is a key component to healthy sleep. As tryptophan cannot be naturally created by the body, it must be obtained through food. Also, the magic combination of melatonin, magnesium, and zinc has been found to work wonders for sleep, so foods or combinations of foods that contain these nutrients can be beneficial.

Sleepy Food Shopping List

The following list is a great starting point for incorporating sleep-inducing foods into your diet. The list is organized based on the nutrients that help with sleep and the foods associated with those nutrients. Incorporate this food into the later hours of your day for maximum benefit.

Foods with Tryptophan

Foods with Melatonin

Foods with Vitamin D and Omega-3 Fatty Acids that Regulate Serotonin

Foods with Magnesium

Foods with Zinc

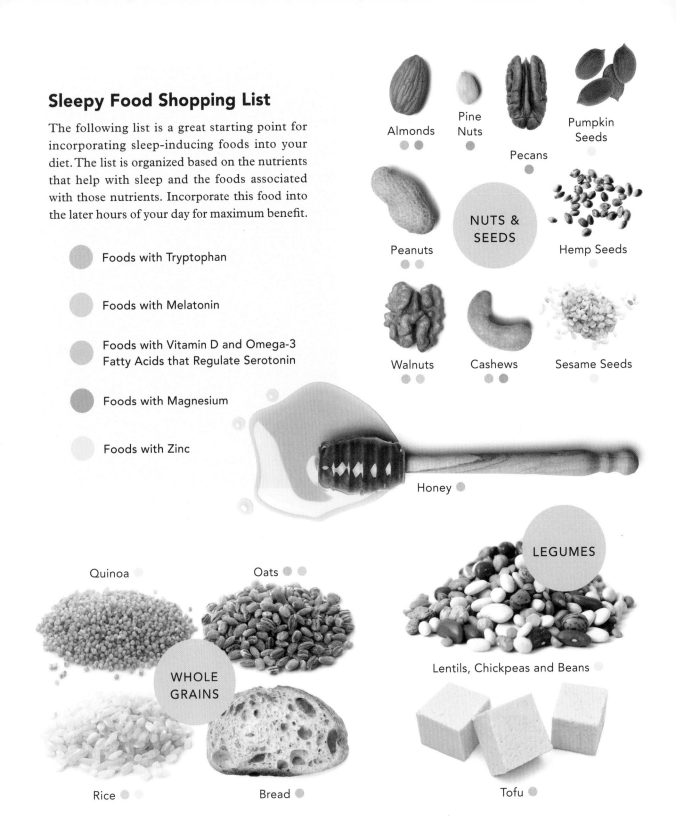

Almonds

Pine Nuts

Pecans

Pumpkin Seeds

NUTS & SEEDS

Peanuts

Hemp Seeds

Walnuts

Cashews

Sesame Seeds

Honey

Quinoa

Oats

WHOLE GRAINS

LEGUMES

Lentils, Chickpeas and Beans

Rice

Bread

Tofu

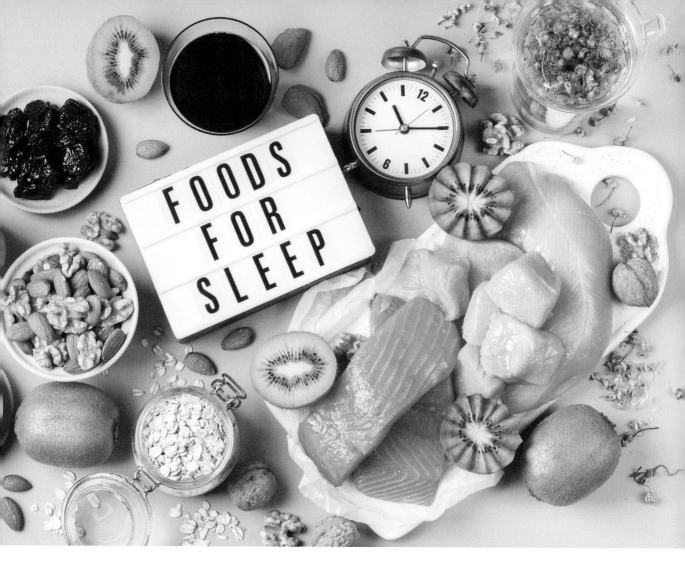

SEAFOOD:

Salmon ● ● ●
Tuna ● ●
Halibut ●
Sardines ●
Anchovies ●
Crab ●
Oysters ●
Shrimp ● ●

MEAT:

Chicken ●
Turkey ●
Beef ●
Lamb ●
Pork ●

FRUIT:

Bananas ● ●
Tart Cherries ●
Avocado ● ●
Kiwi ●
Plums ●
Pineapple ●
Olives ●
Apples ●

VEGETABLES:

Asparagus ●
Tomato ● ●
Potaoes ●
Sweet Potato ●
Spinach ●
Kale ●
Corn ●
Broccoli ●

DAIRY

Milk ●
Eggs ●
Cheese ●

Drinking for Sleep

In addition to the food that you consume, the beverages you drink have an impact on the quality of your sleep.

—

Sugar, alcohol, and caffeine can disrupt your sleep patterns. Avoid sugary drinks in the evening because they can confuse your body and create a false feeling of energy. Though alcohol can help you fall asleep, it will disrupt your ability to stay asleep. Because of this, avoid alcohol for the four to six hours before you get into bed. As caffeine is a stimulant, it can keep you awake and make it very difficult to fall asleep. Caffeine is found in more than your morning coffee; it can be hidden in soda, tea, chocolate, and even certain medications. Avoid caffeine at least six hours before bedtime. If you crave the taste of coffee in the later hours of the day, find a coffee replacement to sip on. Some coffee replacements even contain sleep-enhancing adaptogens.

If you sip on beverages in the evening, stop hydrating two hours before bedtime so that your sleep isn't interrupted by the need to use the restroom.

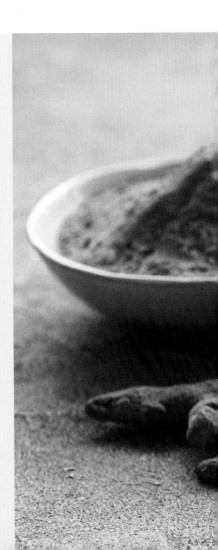

RECIPE

SOOTHING NIGHTTIME BEVERAGES

Malted milk is a simple beverage made by combining malted milk powder - a combination of barley, evaporated milk, and wheat—with milk. This milk is full of sleep-inducing vitamins and minerals like magnesium, zinc, and vitamin B. For a tasty nighttime sip, buy a malted milk powder of your choice and whisk it into a mug of warm milk.

If you're looking for a slightly more involved drink recipe with many healing and sleep benefits, you can make yourself a mug of Golden Milk. This Golden Milk recipe is from the first book in this series, *The Complete Guide to Self Care: Best Practices for a Happier and Healthier You.* Golden Milk is a traditional Indian drink that helps with digestion, is anti-inflammatory, promotes sleep, and is delicious.

To make Golden Milk, add 2 cups of milk or almond milk to a saucepan. Then add 1 ½ teaspoons of turmeric powder, 1 tablespoon coconut oil, and a pinch of black pepper. You can also add 1/2 teaspoon of powdered ginger if you like things a little sweet and spicy. If you like things on the sweeter side, add a dash of honey. Place the saucepan over medium high heat and whisk the ingredients together. Once the liquid begins to simmer, remove the Golden Milk from the stove and transfer it to your favorite mug. Sip slowly and enjoy.

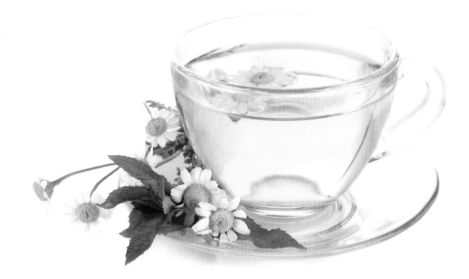

HERBAL TEAS TO HELP YOU FALL ASLEEP AND STAY ASLEEP

Another recommended evening beverage is non-caffinated tea. Herbal teas are a wonderful way to enjoy your tea ritual without the stimulation of caffeine. Two herbal teas that work to facilitate sleep are chamomile tea and lavender tea. You can also find herbal tea blends that are created to assist with sleep. If you would like to elevate your tea drinking experience, you can add a bit of warmed milk and even a dash of honey, as both promote sleep.

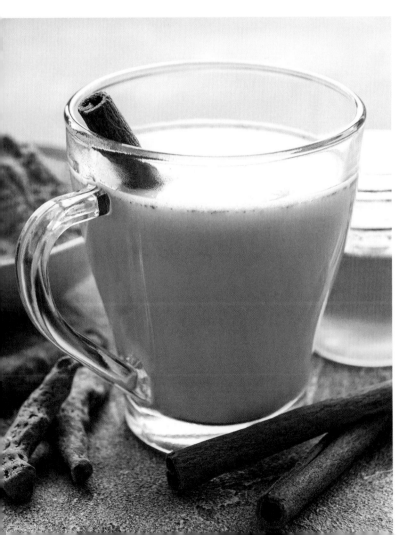

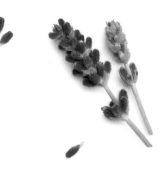

The Perfect Bedtime Ritual

As you are looking to set up a routine, or ritual, that you complete each night before going to bed, incorporate elements that are soothing, relaxing, calming, and signal a feeling of peace and safety so that you can gently drift off to sleep. The following are two kinds of rituals that you can utilize in your bedtime routine.

Evening Water Ritual

Self-soothing is the ability to treat yourself in a way that decreases negative feelings.

To properly self-soothe, find a private, peaceful, and quiet environment. This can be found in the shower or the bath. When you rinse off in the evening, you can incorporate the following elements to assist yourself with self-soothing.

1 **Focus on the temperature of the water in your shower or bath.** Though a hot shower feels great, it can also be too stimulating before bed. Choose a temperature that Goldilocks would approve of: not too hot and not too cold. It should feel slightly warmer than the temperature of your skin. This is your "just right" water temperature.

2 **Allow time for your hair to dry.** If you are going to wash your hair, allocate enough time for your hair to dry before bed. Blow drying your hair is loud, hot, and involves physical movement—all things you want to avoid before bedtime. Going to bed with a wet head is strongly discouraged because the temperature of your hair can disrupt your ability to get steady sleep by impacting your body temperature. A good solution is to invest in a highly absorbent microfiber towel. You can wash your hair, towel dry it, wrap your hair in a microfiber towel for fifteen minutes to allow it to absorb extra water, and then you can take off the towel to let the rest of the moisture in your hair evaporate. If you do not have enough time for your hair to dry, skip washing your hair altogether and make that a daytime activity.

3 **Focus on your environment.** The area where you take your evening shower or bath should be as soothing as possible. For inspiration, think about elements that are included in a spa setting. You can light a candle or play calming music. You can incorporate beautiful plants pieces of art that relaxes you.

4 **Utilize soothing products with aromatherapy benefits.** If you are using products like body wash, shaving cream, shampoo, and conditioner, consider purchasing some products that are specific to your evening routine. A tingly citrus body wash or scalp invigorating shampoo is great during the day, but these stimulating products negatively impact your ability to relax. Instead, think about owning a set of daytime and nighttime products with varying scents. Nighttime products can include soothing, earthy, calming, and relaxing scents. If you want to simplify your routine and only use one set of products, consider investing in unscented products that don't sway your stimulation one way or the other.

5 **Visualize yourself releasing the worries of the day.** This shower is a time for you to clean your body and mind. As you wash away the physical debris of the day, visualize the mental debris of the day—stress, anxiety, negative emotions, or overwhelm —rinsing away with it. Take deep cleansing breaths while you do this. Tell yourself that anything negative that you experienced that day has been washed down the drain. You can even say it aloud at the end of your shower: "*I am clean and clear* both in body and mind. I am ready to rest and restore."

6 **Prioritize your comfort.** Your goal is to maintain the soothing calm that you felt during your shower to help with sleep. The fabrics that touch your skin can help protect the calm you have created. Think of the towel you use to dry off. Can this towel be improved upon? Find a towel that is plush and oversized, so you can wrap yourself up in it. You can also invest in a soft robe and slippers to put on the moment you have finished drying off.

Create Your Own
Wind-down Ritual

When you set out to create your bedtime ritual, think about the things you already do each night before bed. Consider ways you can improve upon those things. Additionally, identify practices you would like to add to your ritual.

For example, if you currently brush your teeth each night and take off your makeup using a makeup wipe before bed, you will want to assess this. When you brush your teeth, could you improve the process by investing in a better toothbrush? Could you swap out your evening toothpaste for something more calming like an herbal toothpaste with chamomile? Instead of using a makeup wipe could you spend an extra minute or two taking off your makeup a different way that is better for your skin and more calming?

Those are the kind of questions you will want to ask yourself to ensure that you have created the very best wind-down ritual or bedtime routine possible.

Following are different suggestions to include in your bedtime ritual. Feel free to incorporate all of the suggestions -—there is nothing wrong with setting aside thirty minutes for yourself to engage in self-care at the end of the day! —or just a few if you want a simplified routine.

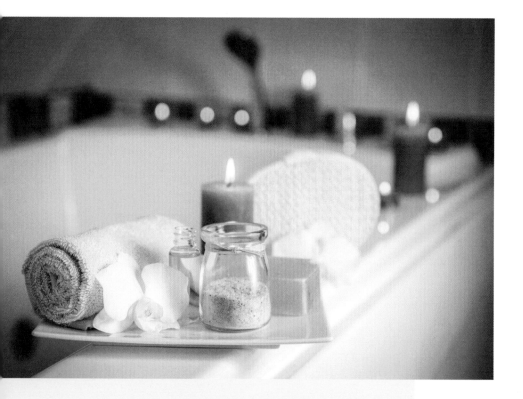

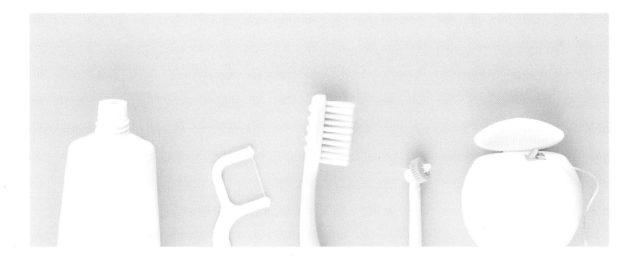

Brushing Your Teeth/Oral Care

Toothbrush: consider upgrading your toothbrush. You can opt for a natural toothbrush that is environmentally friendly and made of sustainable materials like bamboo for a soothing experience. You can also invest in an electric toothbrush if you are seeking a deeper and more efficient way to clean your teeth.

Toothpaste: most toothpastes are minty and bright. The invigorating taste of mint may be too stimulating before bed. Consider purchasing a nighttime toothpaste. This toothpaste can be herbal, it can contain soothing scents for sleep, or it can be a milder flavor that is soothing.

Floss: it is important to floss each day to maintain healthy gums. Healthy gums help your teeth stay strong, which becomes increasingly vital as you age. If you currently do not floss, incorporating nightly flossing into your routine is a great place to start. If you already floss, you may want to find a floss that is better than the current one you are using. Try to find a floss made from natural fibers, like coconut, or lightly flavored with a taste that you enjoy. If you have a difficult time reaching the back corners of your mouth, you may want to try a floss pick. Additionally, leaving your floss out on your counter can remind you of this important part of your routine, so find floss that is beautifully packaged.

Water Flosser: if you do not like traditional flossing, water flossing is a wonderful alternative that provides similar benefits without having to run a piece of waxed string between each tooth. This option is great for people with sensitive or swollen gums or those who have braces. This flosser uses water pressure to remove food and bacteria from between your teeth. You simply fill a reservoir with water and move the device around your gums and mouth. There are many options available with a variety of price points and styles. Find a water flosser that fits your bathroom decor so you can leave it out for easy access.

Tongue Scraper: scraping your tongue can improve the health of your mouth, gums, and teeth. It can also fight bad breath, remove bacteria, and improve your sense of taste. Using a tongue scraper removes 30% more negative elements from the tongue then brushing with a toothbrush alone. It is easy, safe, and quick to scrape your tongue. You can purchase tongue scrapers made from a variety of materials and in a myriad of styles.

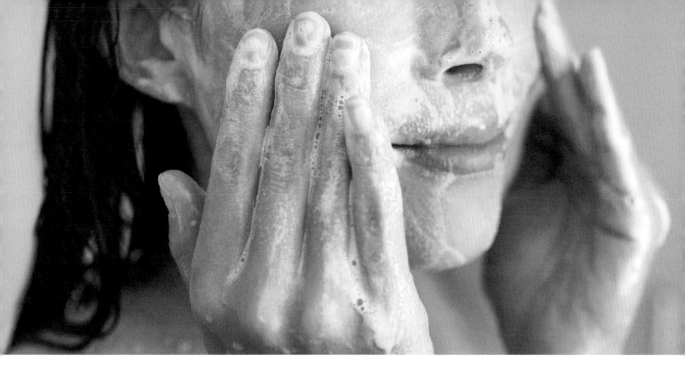

Skincare and Facial Massage

Cleansing: Leaving makeup on your face not only keeps bacteria trapped in the skin, but transfers this bacteria, makeup, and oils to your pillowcase and pillow. Even if you do not wear makeup, you should still clean your face as you have picked up bacteria and pollutants throughout the day from the environment. You do not want your unwashed face to create a breeding ground for sleep-disrupting bacteria.

If you currently use a traditional drugstore cleanser or makeup wipes to remove your makeup, you can upgrade this part of your routine. If you insist on using makeup wipes, find some that are made with clean ingredients and are unscented or scented with something natural and calming.

If you use cleanser to remove your makeup, make the switch to oil cleansing. Oil cleansing works by rubbing your face with oil to break down and remove makeup, reduces the amount of acne-producing oil your skin creates, and cleans out clogged pores. You can buy an oil cleanser or use any of your favorite organic cold-pressed oils - like olive oil, castor oil, jojoba oil, or almond oil. To oil cleanse, take a teaspoon of oil and rub it all over your face in a circular motion for a couple of minutes to allow everything to break down. Then take a washcloth soaked in warm water and use it to gently remove the excess oil and broken-down makeup and bacteria. You can rub any remaining oil into your skin for extra hydration.

For a simple way to cleanse your face and remove makeup with added skin-loving benefits, use micellar water. This French beauty secret looks and feels like water but contains micelles. Micelles are microparticles that trap dirt and makeup and pull them off your face. To use this method of cleansing, soak an organic cotton round with micellar water and gently swipe it across your face. It removes face makeup and is gentle and effective at removing eye makeup, as well. Use a micellar water that is fragrance free. If you want to add a fragrance to the treatment, you can place ten-to-fifteen drops of lavender oil or rose oil into your micellar water.

Skin treatments: if you are currently a rinse-the-makeup-off-and-sleep type, you may want to think about adding some skincare to your nighttime ritual. There are a variety of targeted treatments available that can help you get the skin of your dreams while you dream. Identify your individual skin concerns—acne, aging, lack of elasticity, discoloration, etc. —and search for a product that targets this. Find products that are clean, organic, cruelty-free, and natural when you can. These products are not only better for the earth and the animals, they are better for you. Because your skin is highly absorbent, anything you put on it will end up in your system. Only incorporate one new skincare product at a time to ensure that your skin responds favorably.

Moisturizing: it is common to become dehydrated during sleep. This dehydration impacts your body and organs, including your skin, which is the largest organ you have. To protect your skin against dehydration, you can incorporate a moisturizing component in your routine. Remember, it is not just your face that needs hydration while you sleep. Your neck and chest deserve some extra attention as they are both prone to showing the signs of aging. If the skin on your body feels dry when you wake, you might want to apply a light body lotion or oil to your skin before sleep. Another area that can benefit from extra hydration are your hands and your feet. Use a thick and rich cream on your hands and feet to really lock in moisture and help treat cuticles and calluses.

When it comes to moisturizing your face, you can choose an oil, a gel, or a lotion. Oils are great for most skin types except for those who are highly acne-prone. You can find oil mixtures to purchase or you can simply use some castor oil or marula oil. Gels are great for all skin types, but especially for those with acne-prone skin who are trying to avoid excess oils. Some gel moisturizers can also be used as an overnight mask that you wipe off in the morning. Check the label to see if the gel product

you have chosen can be multi-purposed into a mask. Facial lotions can be used on all skin types and typically state if they are for dry, oily, or combo skin on the label.

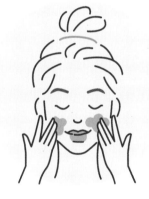

Certain areas of your face might need extra hydration or specialized hydration. This is especially true for your under eyes. The under eye area is delicate and is one of the first to show signs of aging, exhaustion, or dehydration. Under eye creams are formulated specially for the delicate skin around your eye. If you are looking for a homemade under eye remedy, you can keep organic cotton pads soaked in rose water in your fridge and let these sit on your eyes. You can also use a tiny bit of honey underneath your eyes.

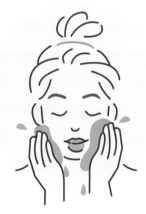

Facial massage: while you apply your oil cleanser, your skin treatments, or your facial moisturizer, you can concurrently indulge in facial massage. To do this, gently tap and massage your face with your fingers. Start at the top near your forehead and work your way down your face constantly moving your fingers from the center of your face to the outside. When you get to your jaw, rub your hands firmly from the sides of your jaw near your ears down the sides of your neck. Do this a few times. This allows the toxins and fluids to drain from your face.

If you want to try another form of facial massage, purchase a facial roller. Facial rolling is an ancient beauty practice that helps detoxify the face by promoting lymphatic drainage. Some other benefits of facial rolling are:

- Defined cheekbones and jawline
- Reduction in under eye circles and puffy eyes
- Clears sinuses
- Decreases tension in the facial muscles
- Fights the signs of aging
- Deeper penetration of skincare products

You can purchase facial rollers made from a variety of materials, but many are made out of crystals like rose quartz or jade. If you believe in the healing power of crystals - or you just find them to be beautiful - look for an amethyst facial roller. Amethyst is a purple semi-precious stone that is believed to soothe stress, promote relaxation, decrease anxiety, and increase the clarity of your dreams.

Lip scrub: the skin on your lips can dry out, peel, and crack. You can purchase a lip scrub online or make a simple one at home by combining a little bit of skin-safe and food-safe oil — like olive oil or almond oil—with a natural exfoliant like sugar. Take a little bit of the lip scrub and rub it in a circular motion with your finger. Remove with a warm damp cloth. Do not scrub your lips every night as this can be too much on the delicate skin. Aim for incorporating this into your wind-down ritual once or twice a week.

Lip mask: if you scrub your lips, an overnight lip mask is non-negotiable. Newly exposed skin needs extra protection and hydration. It is important to note that this is a great step to incorporate to protect your lips even if you do not use a lip scrub. Overnight lip masks are easy to apply and foolproof. Put a generous layer of the mask on your lips as the last step in your skincare routine. Your body will absorb the moisture overnight and you will wake to hydrated, plump, and smooth lips.

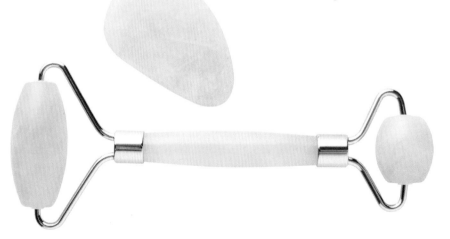

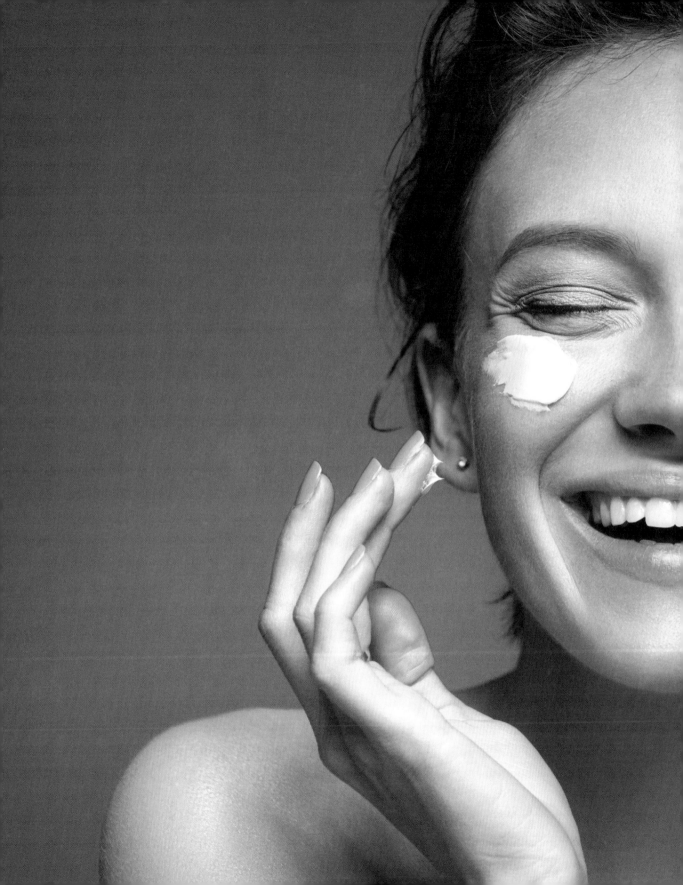

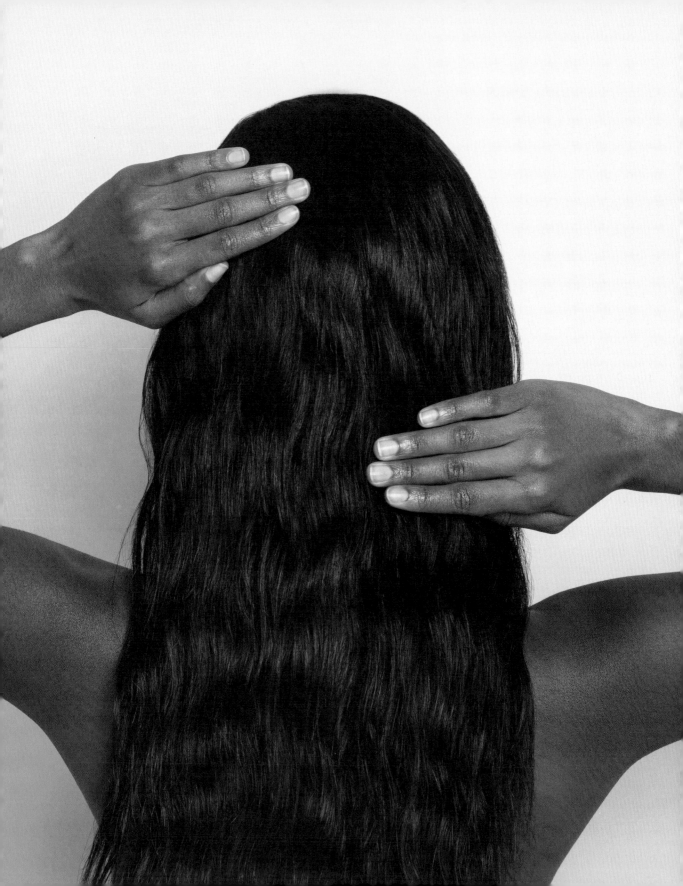

Haircare

Hairbrush: thirty seconds of brushing your hair at night has a host of beauty benefits. Brushing your hair helps distribute the oils evenly which can help with hair health, strength, shine, and can diminish frizz. You likely already own a hairbrush, but is it the ideal brush for hair health? If you use a natural boar bristle hair brush it will gently untangle your hair. It also works the best for distributing healthy scalp oils.

Leave-In Conditioner or a Hair Mask: if your hair is prone to drying out, if you chemically treat or color your hair, or if you're looking for extra shine, apply a leave-in conditioner before sleep to deeply treat your hair. As an added benefit, you can seek out a conditioner that has aromatherapy benefits so that the scents can lull you to sleep. If you need a little more hydration, try an overnight hair mask. There are many formulas available to address different hair concerns. For the simplest and most natural overnight treatment, apply a little bit of argan oil to the ends of your hair and then smooth the rest that is left on your hands over your remaining hair before tying your hair back.

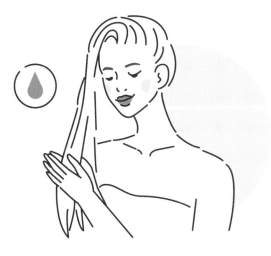

Hair elastic: tie your hair back while you sleep for comfort, so your hair doesn't disrupt your sleep, so any products on your hair stay off your face, and to keep your hair from absorbing your skincare products. If you use hair elastics that contain metal, get rid of them now. Metal causes hair to become damaged and break. It can be made even worse if you are tossing and turning throughout the night; this can cause the metal part of the hair elastic to snag your hair. At night, opt for a wrapped elastic that is coated to prevent hair damage. You can also use a scrunchie. To elevate this experience, purchase silk scrunchies that are aesthetically pleasing and offer hair protection.

When tying your hair back, do not make the mistake of tying your hair back tightly. This can lead to hair damage, headaches, and discomfort that interrupt sleep. A couple easy options are wrapping your hair in a bun and loosely securing your hair on top of your head or putting your hair in a loose braid.

Silk headwrap: these wraps are ideal for people with curly hair to protect their hair and their hairstyle while they sleep. These wraps have other uses, as well. If you are wearing an overnight hair treatment, they can protect the treatment from getting on your pillowcase and help the treatment absorb deeper. Headwraps can help your hair from getting caught, tangled, or damaged while you move in your sleep. They can also help preserve a hairstyle like braids or curls. Additionally, silk head wraps come in a variety of patterns and colors so they add a fun element of style to your nighttime ritual.

Yoga and Meditation

Yoga is an ancient practice that combines body posturing and movement, breath, and meditation. This holistic practice focuses on the mind-body connection. Yoga involves a series of poses or postures that are held by the body for a period of time while keeping your mind present.

There are many benefits to yoga, both for the body and for the mind.

PHYSICAL BENEFITS OF YOGA
- Strengthens muscles
- Relieves aches and pains
- Reduces inflammation
- Increases heart health

MENTAL AND EMOTIONAL BENEFITS OF YOGA
- Reduces stress and anxiety
- Elevates mood
- Increases clarity
- Assists with sleep

Learning yoga is more accessible than ever before. You can choose to learn yoga the traditional way. You may want to attend a yoga class or receive training from a yoga instructor. If you would like to go at it on your own, you can look up online yoga classes, use an app on your smartphone that walks you through yoga, or start with the simple positions in the Moon Flow Exercise below.

Meditation is sitting or lying down comfortably in stillness with your eyes closed while breathing deeply. During meditation, you focus on your breath, allow your thoughts to appear without judgment, acknowledge and release your thoughts, and return to focusing on your breath. This allows you to understand the thoughts that are running through your subconscious. This self-awareness allows you to become more intentional and present in your life.

Meditation is a practice that many people find challenging. Contrary to what you may have heard, you cannot be "bad" at meditating. If you think you are meditating incorrectly because you have racing thoughts, feel restless, cannot seem to stay present or focused, or continually get distracted try to remind yourself that this is normal and the exact reason you are meditating. These modern maladies, or these sources of brain chaos, are very common in humans today and meditation - with repeated practice and dedication - assists you with battling this mental overwhelm. The key is to begin a consistent meditation practice. It is known as a practice because it is something that you are literally *practicing*. The continuation of this practice will allow you to grow and shift and your meditation skills expand.

There are many benefits to meditation. Similar to yoga, this practice has benefits for the mind and the body.

PHYSICAL BENEFITS OF MEDITATION
- Decreases the risk of heart disease
- Helps to manage pain
- Assists with weight management

MENTAL AND EMOTIONAL BENEFITS OF MEDITATION
- Creates positive thinking patterns
- Reduces stress and aggression
- Decreases irritability
- Assists with the management of depression
- Reduces feelings of anxiety
- Increases relaxation
- Enhances clarity and focus
- Assists with sleep

There are many ways to learn about meditation. If you would like to learn meditation from a practitioner, you can seek out a meditation guide to assist you or attend a meditation class. If you would like to learn about meditation from the comfort of your own home, you can take a guided meditation class online or even download a meditation app to your smartphone. Additionally, you can attempt meditation on your own by doing the following exercise.

MEDITATION BASICS

If you would like to practice meditation on your own, here is a short introduction:

(2) **Find a secluded spot where you can sit comfortably. You can participate in this practice in silence, or you can choose to play some calming music.** If you choose to listen to music, choose something instrumental or ambient. You can find free meditation playlists easily online or you can make your own.

(2) **Settle in so that you feel as comfortable as possible.** Close your eyes and begin to breathe slowly, deeply, and intentionally. Breathe in through your nose and out of your mouth. Feel the breath enter your lungs. If you are breathing deeply while relaxed, you will feel your belly rise and fall with your breath.

(2) **Follow or track your breath. In.** Out. Follow the air as it makes its way through your nose, all the way down into your lungs and belly, and then as it travels back upward to exit your body out of your mouth. Keep breathing and tracking your breath slowly and rhythmically.

(2) **If a thought or feeling pops up that distracts you from focusing on your breath, acknowledge the thought without judgment.** Then release it. This can be difficult to do. Imagine yourself as a passive observer of your thoughts who is not directly connected to them. Give the thought a moment of attention. Then let it go. Bring your attention back to your breath.

So this makes sense, here is an example. *You are meditating and focusing on following your breath. You begin to feel peaceful, calm, and centered. All of a sudden you think about what you need to make for dinner. You step back in your mind's eye to observe the thought. Your internal observer thinks, "Hmm, I just thought about what I need to make for dinner. That is what was present*

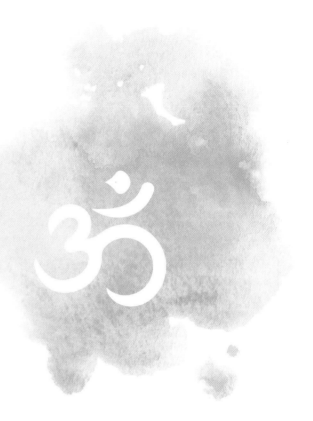

in my mind. I choose to release that thought. All I have to do right now is be exactly where I am focusing on my breath." And then you refocus on your breath and continue to meditate.

Note: Having thoughts during meditation is completely normal. Instead of viewing the time spent acknowledging your thoughts as a setback, shift your perspective. Every thought that pops up and that you acknowledge is something new you have learned about your internal programming. The more you learn about yourself, the better you can be.

(2) **Continue to repeat steps 3 and 4.** You can practice for five minutes, thirty minutes, or even an hour. There is no set amount of time to devote to your practice. Just keep practicing for optimum results!

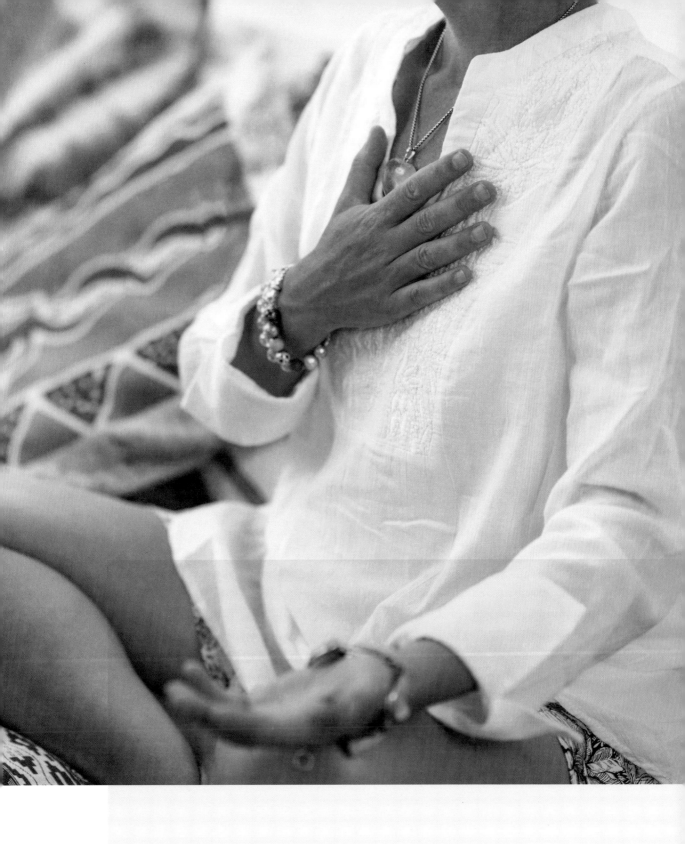

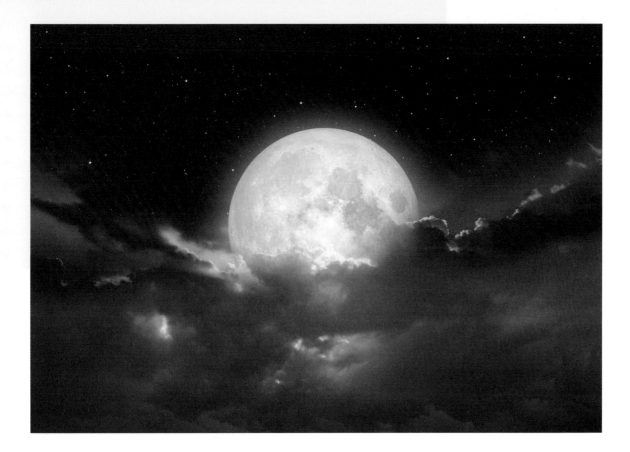

Intention Setting and the Phases of the Moon

Intention setting is the practice of committing to a thought or desire that is clearly defined coupled with the willingness to act to make that desire manifest. Basically, it's identifying something you want to achieve and committing yourself to making it happen. The key is to phrase it as if it has already happened. This helps the concept cement itself into your brain as more than a possibility; instead, you will see it as a reality.

EXAMPLES OF INTENTIONS

- *I am honest in my words and actions.*
- *I exercise patience with my co-workers.*
- *I prioritize my healthy sleep habits.*

As it can be difficult for some people to come up with a clear intention or even know where to begin, it can be helpful to have a method to keep you inspired and on track. One such method is using the moon to guide your intention-setting practice.

Yes, the moon. It might sound a little woo-woo to you (or it might not!), but the moon can serve as a kind of intention setting calendar in the sky.

Here's how: the moon goes through eight phases each 28-day lunar cycle. For those with a spiritual interest in the moon, each moon phase is thought to connect with a different theme. Even without a connection to the moon, knowing the phases of the moon and their correlating themes can inspire your intention for meditation or to give you something to focus on during your yoga flow.

The Eight Phases of the Moon and Their Corresponding Themes

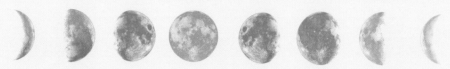

NEW MOON: this is a time when the moon is not visible in the sky. Use this time of darkness to set an intention about things in your life that you want to be brought into the light.
Intention Example: *I have clarity in who I am and what I want.*

WAXING CRESCENT: a sliver of moon appears in the sky. The moon is growing. This is a time for you to set an intention about your personal growth.
Intention Example: *I am open to constructive criticism and self-improvement.*

FIRST QUARTER: the moon will be perfectly illuminated on one half. It looks like there is a solid boundary between the light and dark side of the moon. This is a time to set an intention connected to a boundary you would like to set or a clear decision you would like to make.
Intention Example: *I set clear boundaries as to how I spend my time and who I spend it with.*

WAXING GIBBOUS: the moon is more than half full of light, but not yet all the way full. Set an intention to get clarity on any adjustments you want to make to help you reach your fullest potential.
Intention Example: *I am open to change and adjust my course easily.*

FULL MOON: the moon is now a bright white orb in the sky full of light. You can set an intention to illuminate what is working for you and against you in your life.
Intention Example: *Intention Example: I pour my energy into the elements assisting me in my life and block my energy from anything hindering me.*

WANING GIBBOUS: the moon's light begins to lessen and appears much like the waxing gibbous, but in reverse. The moon achieved its fullest potential. This is a time to set an intention involving gratitude.
Intention Example: *I am grateful for my physical and mental health.*

THIRD QUARTER: this moon is a mirror image of the first quarter moon. The light only fills half of the moon at this point. Set an intention about what you would like to release in your life.
Intention Example: *I release the anger I felt toward my friend; I forgive her.*

WANING CRESCENT: the moon is a tiny sliver in the sky about to enter a period of total darkness. The moon is preparing for a period of rest. Set an intention involving rest and regeneration.
Intention Example: *I allow myself ample time to rest and heal.*

Moon Flow Exercise

This exercise combines all of the concepts explained in this section: yoga, meditation, intention setting, and the phases of the moon. You can do this exercise on any evening you wish to prepare for sleep. You can continue to repeat this exercise nightly if it resonates with you.

① **Identify the moon phase.** You can do this by stepping outside and looking up at the moon or performing a quick internet search. There are also apps that track the phase of the moon.

② **Set your corresponding intention.** Look to the phases above to find the corresponding intention-setting theme. Create an intention for yourself based on this theme.

③ **Find a comfortable place.** Get settled into a comfortable position. Once you feel settled in, state the intention you created for yourself aloud. This sets the tone for the meditation and yoga flow to follow.

④ **Meditate for ten minutes.** Follow the steps listed above to meditate on your own or use a guided meditation app. You can choose to play music or sit in silence.

⑤ **Yoga flow for ten minutes.** This gentle flow can be done using a mat placed near a wall or on your bed if it rests against a wall. Remember to breathe deeply and close your eyes throughout the practice.

Start by lying down on your mat or the bed, flat on your back, with your head away from the wall and your feet towards the wall.

The first pose you will enter is **Corpse Pose** *(Savasana)*. Allow your arms and legs to settle comfortably out toward your sides as you lie on your back. Remain in this position for 1 minute.

You will now transition to **Reclining Butterfly Pose** *(Supta Baddha Konasana)*. To do this, slowly bring your knees out to the sides of your body, and bring the bases of your feet together. Once your feet are together, your legs should form a kind of diamond. Breathe deeply, and place one hand on your stomach and the other hand on your heart. Remain in this position for 2 minutes.

You will now transition to the **Legs-Up-the-Wall Pose** *(Viparita Karani)*. Shift your hips close to the wall and raise your legs up against the wall. If you can keep your legs straight without much resistance, do so. Bend your knees if you feel tightness or discomfort. Extend your arms out to your sides with your palms up. If you find you need to support your spine or lower back, feel free to use a blanket as a makeshift bolster for support. Remain in this position for 4 minutes.

You will now transition back to **Reclining Butterfly Pose** for 2 minutes.

At the end of the 2 minutes, you will transition back to the **Corpse Pose** for 1 minute.

At the end of your flow, speak your intention aloud again.

⑥ **Prepare for sleep.** Your body and mind should now feel centered, relaxed, and ready for a night of rest.

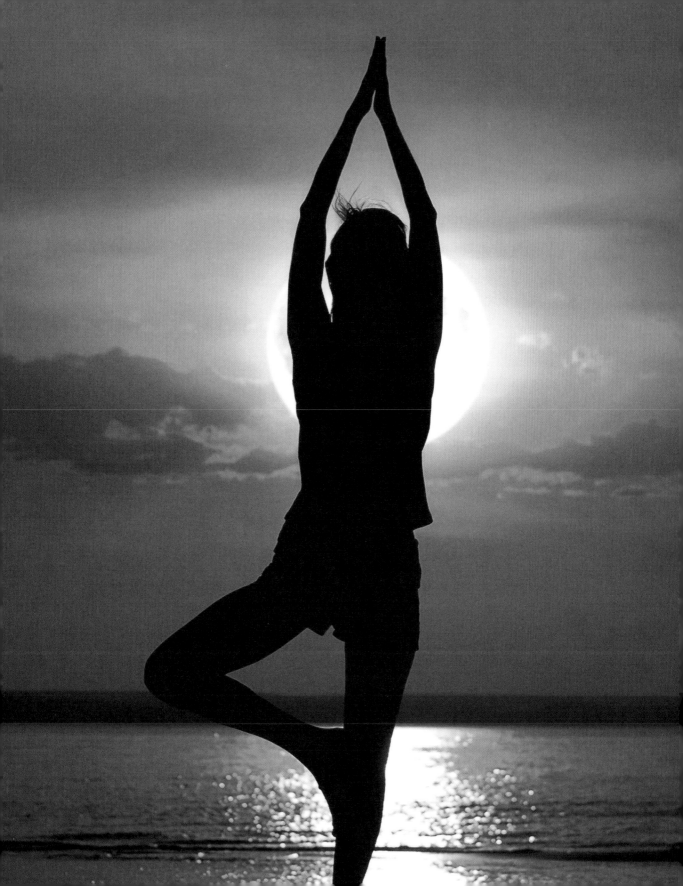

Breathwork

Breathwork refers to breathing practices which are believed to be therapeutic in nature. These practices last anywhere from a few minutes to an hour and involve timing the breath. You can time breathing in and out, holding your breath, or both. It is believed that breathwork helps people get to the mental state they are seeking when meditating, but much faster. In fact, breathwork can help detach you from your thoughts entirely which can allow healing and relaxation to occur at a swift pace.

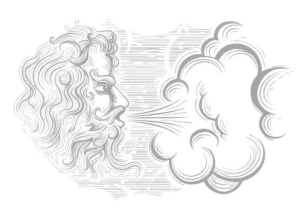

The practice can be for the benefit of the body, the mind, or the emotions. Some people utilize this practice to mitigate trauma while others use it to relax, release, and feel present.

BENEFITS OF BREATHWORK

- Reduces stress
- Lowers blood pressure
- Releases trauma
- Increases immunity
- Increases joy
- Processes emotions

You can learn to practice breathwork in a variety of ways. Much like yoga and meditation, you can choose to find a breathwork teacher or attend a class or workshop. You can also find courses and guided breathwork sessions online. There are apps that you can download that help you create your own breathwork routine. Additionally, you can research the practice online and create your own breathwork practice.

Breathwork is beneficial for sleep because it allows you to release the stressors of the day. It can bring you to a centered and present place, which helps to reduce depression and anxiety. It can also bring you to a clear-headed space, which is an ideal mindset for restful sleep.

When you begin your practice, listen to your body. Everyone has a different experience with breathwork. For some it is mild and for others it can be a total mind-body experience. When you first start your breathwork journey, it is important to practice in a safe place while lying down. This is vital because many people get light-headed or experience tingling or chills when they begin their practice. If, at any time, breathwork feels straining on the body or mind, take a break.

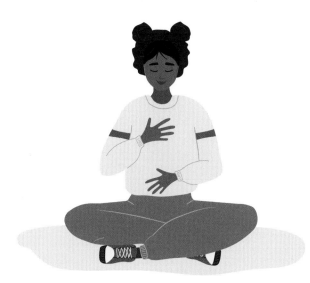

BREATHING FOR BEGINNERS

To begin your breathwork practice, start by learning to breathe deeply and to use your breath for relaxation. This is a wonderful practice to do in the evening to prepare for sleep.

(5) **Find a quiet spot.** You can choose to partake in this practice in silence or you can play music. This can be any relaxing music of your choice.

(5) **Lie down somewhere comfortable where you can fully stretch out.** This can be on a couch, on your bed, or on a mat.

(5) **Place your hands lightly on top of your belly.**

(5) **Breathe in deeply through your nose for a count of 4.** Bring the breath down into the belly. Watch your belly rise and feel it fill up with air.

(5) **Exhale out of your mouth for a count of 8.** Continue to do this for ten minutes.

(5) **At the end of the practice, take note of how you feel.** Are your limbs more relaxed? Do you feel more present and aware? Does your mind feel clear? Did you release some stress in your body and mind? Do you feel ready to sleep.

Count and Breathe Yourself to Sleep

This controlled breathing exercise is perfect for those nights when you lie down, close your eyes, and cannot fall asleep. Instead of counting sheep, try counting your breath. This commonly recommended 4-7-8 breath practice allows your body to slow down, relaxes the pace of your heart, and helps release anxiety.

(1) In your bed with the lights off, comfortably lie on your back. You can keep the pillow under your head for this exercise because, ideally, you will drift off to sleep before you complete it!

(2) Place your hands on your belly or rest your arms gently to your sides. Relax your arms and legs.

(3) With your eyes closed, breathe in through your nose for the count of 4. Visualize this breath making its way all the way down to your belly.

(4) Gently hold this breath for the count of 7.

(5) Release this breath for the count of 8.

(6) Repeat this cycle for ten minutes or until you fall asleep. If you are not asleep or ready for sleep at the end of the ten minutes, you can repeat this practice again.

Taming Anxiety

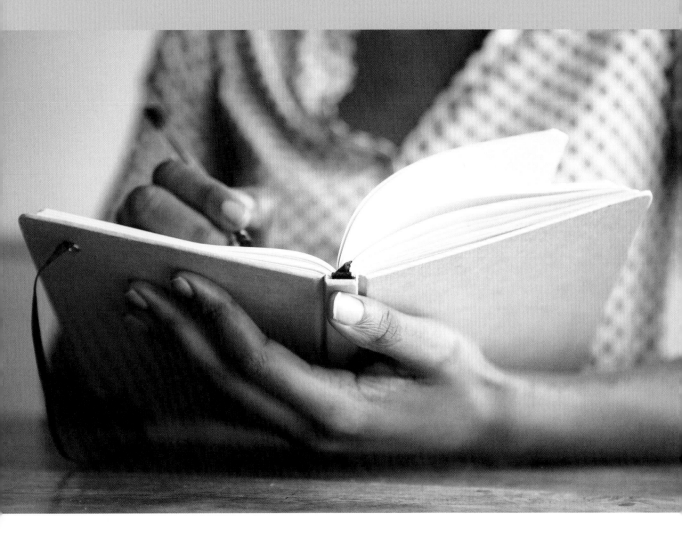

How to Get it Out of Your Head and Onto the Page

If you have ever experienced racing thoughts, restlessness, a rapid heartbeat paired with stress, or feelings of fear or worry that you cannot seem to control, you've likely had a bout of anxiety. Anxiety is a normal and healthy part of life, but that doesn't mean you should allow it to negatively impact you.

The negative impacts of anxiety tend to be felt in conjunction with the experience of anxiety. While you are feeling anxious, your body engages its fight or flight response, which causes physical and mental changes in your body. You may find it hard to get a deep breath or it may feel like your heart is racing.

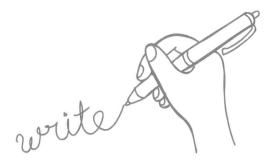

You might get nauseous. You may find it difficult to fall asleep, stay asleep, or you may be chronically exhausted. Anxiety can also cause your muscles to cramp and your immune system to crash.

Anxiety can come and go with the stressors of life; this is considered normal anxiety. If your anxiety is more constant, it can become an anxiety disorder. If you have a medical anxiety disorder, you are not alone. Forty million people in the United States have anxiety disorders. To put this another way, it is estimated that 19.1% of adults experience an anxiety disorder each year and ⅓ of adults have an anxiety disorder at some point in their life. Regardless of the kind of anxiety you are experiencing—the normal run-of-the-mill kind of anxiety or a full-fledged anxiety disorder—there are coping mechanisms and strategies to fight this internal foe.

It should be noted that if you believe that you have an anxiety disorder—meaning that your feelings of anxiety interfere with your daily life frequently—you should seek medical care. Talk therapy is a great place

to start to get clarity on your condition, to receive an appropriate diagnosis, and to gain access to an even bigger toolbox of emotional coping mechanisms.

This section contains a variety of strategies and mechanisms to combat anxiety with a specific focus on relieving anxiety before sleep. Each individual is different and you may find that you benefit from one exercise more than another or that you benefit from a combination of the ideas below.

EXERCISE

Create a Dump Journal

A "dump journal" is exactly what it sounds like: a place to dump your thoughts. This journal exists as a place for you to give those racing thoughts in your head a home so that they stop demanding the valuable real estate in your mind.

What You Need:

An empty journal

A pen you enjoy writing with

① **Keep your dump journal and your pen near your bed.** If you have a bedside table with a drawer, this is a great place to keep it.

② **Set a timer for ten minutes.**

③ **Start the timer and begin to write in your dump journal.** This is a place for you to write the things that are bugging you, worrying you, making you angry, causing you fear, or those things that make you feel overwhelmed or out of control. If it's in your mind and it bugs you, get it out onto the page.

④ **Write continuously for ten minutes.** Do not force yourself to make complete sentences. There may be a word, a person's name, a phrase, or even an image of something that is in your mind. Write it down. Draw it. It doesn't matter how you get it out. It only has to make sense to you.

Drift Off with Thoughts of Gratitude

Another way to negate anxiety, which tends to be associated with a looping thought pattern of negativity, is to replace negativity with positivity. One of the most powerful forms of positive thinking is gratitude. Incorporating a gratitude practice into your nightly routine can a beautiful way to enhance not only your sleep health, but your whole life.

When you shift your focus to a space of positivity by giving thanks, you dedicate your brainpower to it. This, in turn, takes your brain power away from your negative thought loop and redirects it to your positive thoughts. With time, you can train your brain to choose positive thoughts over negative thoughts.

What You Need:

A beautiful journal

A pen you love to write with

① **Keep your gratitude journal out where you can see it and within reach of your bed.**

② **Get into bed, and open your gratitude journal.** You can play some soothing or relaxing music at this time if that enhances your experience.

③ **Turn to a fresh page, and write the date at the top.**

④ **List three things that you are grateful for, and explain why you are grateful for them.** These things can be people, places, things, ideas, experiences, or anything you like. *There are no rules*; this is about what you feel grateful for in your life.

Examples:

- *I am grateful for my sister. She is always there for me to talk to anytime day or night. It feels really good knowing that I have someone I can count on.*

- *I am grateful for my physical health. I do not have any aches or pains, I am able to walk anywhere I please, and I enjoy the feeling of using my body.*

- *I am grateful for good food. I love knowing that pizza and pasta and ice cream exist. I am so happy that I have access to so many different kinds of foods. I even get to go to the farmer's market each week if I want to!*

⑤ **After you are done writing, close your journal and say, "I am so thankful for...".** Finish this sentence with the three things you chose to acknowledge that day.

⑥ **As you turn off the light and lie down for the night, reflect on how grateful you are.** Specifically think about the three things you chose to acknowledge in your journal.

⑦ **Repeat this practice nightly for the most sustained benefits for your mindset.** Do not feel like you need to come up with new things to be grateful for each day; you can write about the same thing for nights on end if it fills your heart with thanks.

Note: this journal is great to have nearby because you can read it anytime you are feeling down or anxious to remind yourself of all the beautiful things in your life.

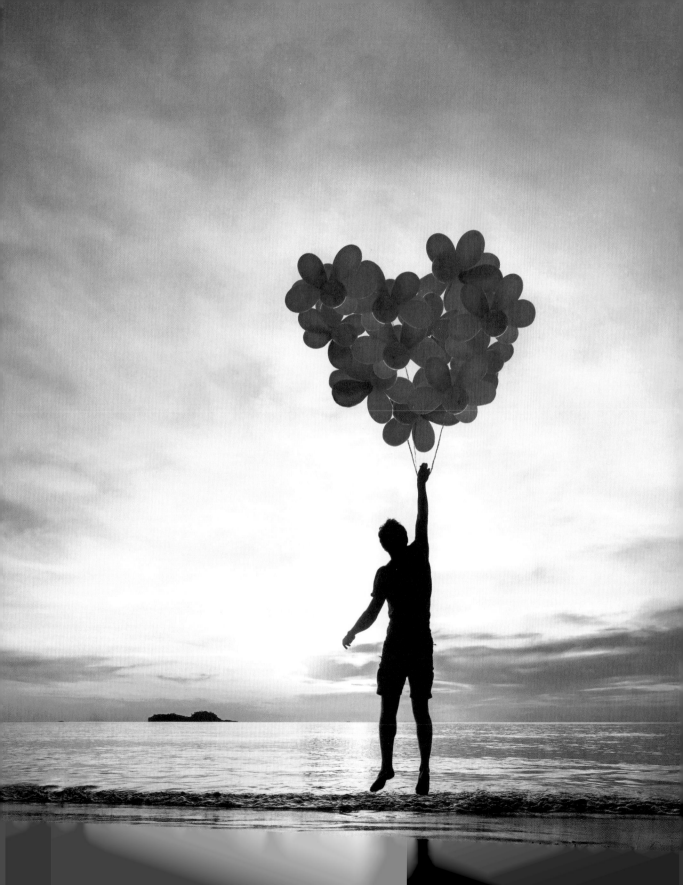

Answer Your Anxiety

This exercise requires emotional maturity. If you feel ready to confront the things that are making you anxious, then this exercise is for you. If reading that feels too daunting, trust your instinct. Focus on the two aforementioned exercises for a month or two and revisit this exercise. If you feel ready then, proceed. If you still don't feel ready, listen to yourself and give yourself more time. Each person's emotional and mental journey is wholly unique; do not put judgment on yourself for your individual needs.

Perform this exercise a couple of hours before bedtime to give yourself time to process. You will be engaging in an internal discussion with yourself and questioning your own thought process and patterns. This can help you gain objectivity when an anxious thought or pattern appears. This can also assist you with keeping yourself calm, relaxed, and clear.

What You Need:

Some pieces of paper

A pen

Scissors

① **Sit somewhere comfortably with a surface to write on.** Do this exercise outside of the bedroom because it may stir up some negative emotions that should not be associated with your space of rest and rejuvenation.

② **Place the piece of paper in front of you, fold it lengthwise, and then unfold it.** The line on the paper should make two long columns: one on the left and one on the right.

③ **In the left hand column, write something you are worried about and the *worst possible scenario* that can occur in this situation.** This is forcing you to identify what your anxiety is telling you —as anxiety is a master at convincing you that the outcome will be dire—and putting it onto the page.

④ **Repeat this for anything that you currently view as a stressor.** Pull out more pieces of paper and repeat the process if needed.

⑤ **Stand up from the table, and walk away from the paper.** Take three deep breaths: in through your nose, down into your belly, and out through your mouth. Now shake out your arms and legs. This gives you time to disconnect from the feelings of anxiety and negativity you were just confronting and give you space to revisit them from a different perspective.

⑥ **Sit back down in front of the paper.** Take three deep breaths, and prepare to confront your thoughts.

⑦ **Address each item you wrote in the left hand column one at a time.** Read what you wrote in the left hand column. Directly across from it in the right hand column, write the *best possible scenario* that can occur in the situation.

⑧ **Continue to do this for each item in the left hand column.** You are essentially entering into a debate with your anxiety where you are choosing a different opinion as to what you believe the outcome will be.

An example of what your sheet might look like:

I'M WORRIED ABOUT:	BEST POSSIBLE SCENARIO:
My annual work review is approaching. I know my boss doesn't like me. I'm going to get a horrible review. Then I will be fired. No one else will hire me, and I won't be able to afford to pay my bills. I'll probably end up homeless.	My annual work review is approaching. I feel like my boss doesn't like me, but she's probably going through things in her own life that I've been taking personally. I know I'm a hard worker, and I give my best. My work review will reflect this. I deserve to be recognized for my efforts, and I know that there are many different businesses who would be happy to have me as an employee.
My best friend has been distant lately. I haven't heard from her. She is bored with our friendship and wants to move on. I will never be able to keep a friend.	My best friend has been distant lately. I'm going to reach out to her and let her know she's been on my mind, and I want to make sure she's doing okay. She probably has something going on in her life and, as her best friend, I'm happy to step up and offer my support. If she doesn't need my support, that's okay, too. I'm a wonderful friend and a very caring person and there are plenty of other friendships out there for me to explore.

(9) After you are done filling in the right hand column, separate the left side from the right side. Use your scissors to cut down the center line. Do this for each piece of paper you wrote on.

(10) Take the left side of the paper and say aloud, "I do not engage in negative thought patterns about my life." Tear the piece of paper into tiny pieces and throw it away.

(11) Take the right side of the paper and say aloud, "This is my truth. I think about my life positively and with hope." Then read everything you wrote on the right side aloud.

(12) When you get into bed, read the right side of the paper again. Keep it on your bedside table. Turn off the lights and continue thinking about the *best possible outcome* of your life until you fall asleep.

Visualization

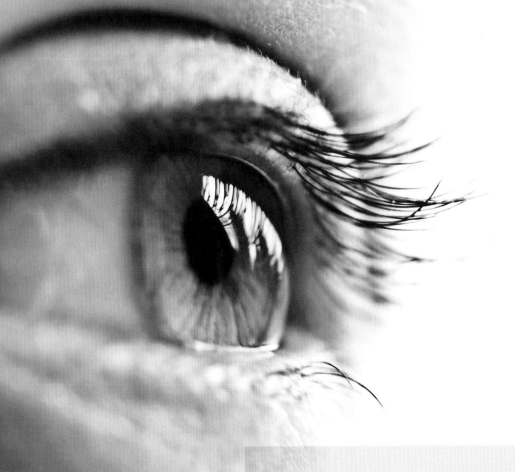

Visualization is another powerful tool that you can add to your get-to-sleep-and-stay-asleep toolbox. Visualization is using your mind's eye to imagine something vividly. It can help you create escapes or safe places in your mind that you can visit anytime.

Using Visualization to Fall Asleep Faster

Visualization is an especially powerful practice when you are seeking sleep. The process of focusing on something lovely engages your brain, while simultaneously relaxing it. This allows your mind to stop engaging with the stressors of the day, to focus on something beautiful, and to soothe itself to sleep.

—

The three following visualizations are guided visualizations. To practice a visualization below, you can do the following:

- Read the visualization in entirety before attempting it and use your recollection to walk yourself through it.

- Record your own voice reading the visualization slowly and at a pace that works for you (you can do this on your phone, computer, or recorder). This allows your mind to be guided by your own voice. This powerful association can assist you with creating your own calming internal voice.

All of these visualizations should be done after you are ready for bed, are comfortably tucked in, and have your eyes closed.

EMPTY ROOM VISUALIZATION

1. **Visualize yourself in an empty room.** This room has nothing on the walls and no furniture in it. Even though the room is bare, you feel overwhelmingly safe and calm in the space. Nothing can hurt you. Nothing can interfere. This is your special space.

2. **Imagine a large cozy chair appearing in the room.** Visualize yourself sitting in this chair. You feel how comfortable it is against your body. You feel completely supported. Spend some time relaxing in this chair and breathing deeply.

3. **Now imagine a big window appearing on one of the walls that your chair is facing.** It fills almost the entire wall. You are able to sit in your comfortable chair feeling safe in your special space, but you can now look outside. The vista that you are looking at is the most beautiful you have ever seen. There are fields of flowers swaying softly in the breeze as far as the eye can see. Pink and purple clouds move slowly across the sky. The sun's rays are gently shining as it begins to set.

4. **Sit and observe this landscape from the comfort of your chair.** Feel free to change the landscape at any time. This is your visualization. You can visualize a tropical beach or snowy mountain peaks or a peaceful lake. All you have to do is visualize something that you find beautiful and imagine it in as much detail as possible.

5. **Do this for as long as you need to prepare yourself for sleep or until you fall asleep.**

STARRY NIGHT VISUALIZATION

① **Visualize yourself lying on your back in a large beautiful field at night while looking up at the stars.** Imagine a warm night time breeze comfortably grazing your skin.

② **Now focus on that sky full of stars. Visualize more stars than you have ever seen.** The stars are bright, clear, white pinpricks of light scattered across the inky sky. Some dots of light are brighter and bigger than the others. These stars are closer to you. Other stars are small and harder to see. These stars must be very far away.

③ **Visualize a meteor shower beginning. Shooting stars begin to appear, one at a time.** Slowly at first and then with increasing frequency. Notice each shooting star. Notice the bright white trail of shimmer that it briefly leaves behind before it seems to be absorbed into the dark of night. Allow yourself to observe the incredible beauty of this.

④ **Wish on the shooting stars. As you continue to watch the shooting stars, you remember that some people believe you should "wish upon a shooting star."** Begin to wish, earnestly and from your heart, for all the things you desire on each star you see. Know in your heart of hearts that all of these wishes will come true. After all, who has ever been blessed with such a meteor shower before?

⑤ **Do this for as long as you need to prepare yourself for sleep or until you fall asleep.**

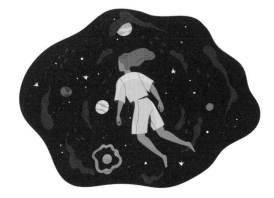

FLOAT AWAY VISUALIZATION

① **Visualize yourself sitting in an innertube in a very peaceful lazy river.** The water is comfortable on your skin.

② **Allow yourself to float gently down the river.** As you begin to float, slowly and safely down the river, it occurs to you that you have nothing more to do than enjoy the feeling of the water on your skin and the beauty of the nature around you.

③ **Imagine looking around and noticing the clear water and the lush banks. You notice deer approaching the river with you in it with no fear and drinking from the pure water.** You see trees and flowers, birds and bunnies, soft rays of sunshine and blue sky. You take your time to feel grateful for each of these things.

④ **As you continue to float, a white butterfly joins you. This butterfly continues with you down the river.** The butterfly is not afraid of you and wants to experience the path of your floating journey by flying around you. You watch the butterfly leave your side, only occasionally, to perch on one of the countless colorful flowers on the river's edge and then to join you again as you float down the river.

⑤ **Do this for as long as you need to prepare yourself for sleep or until you fall asleep.**

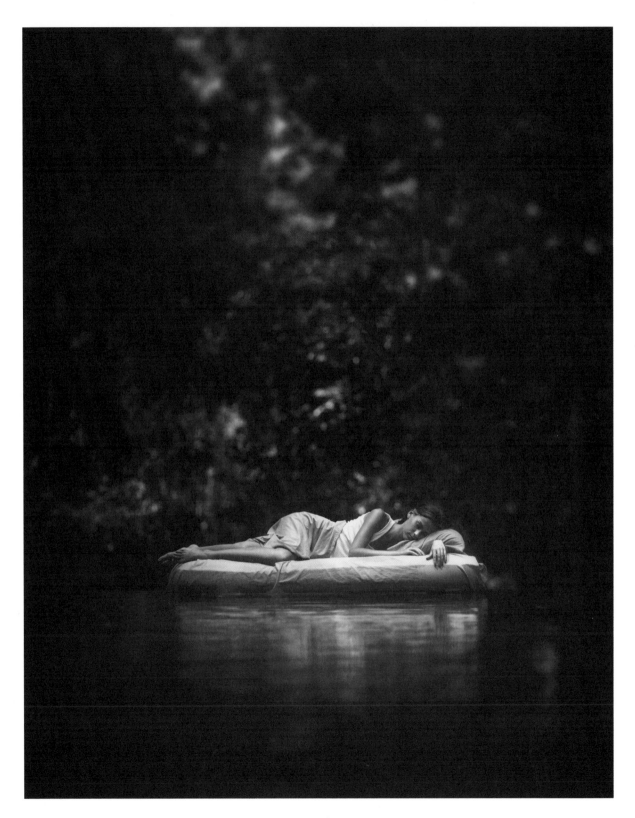

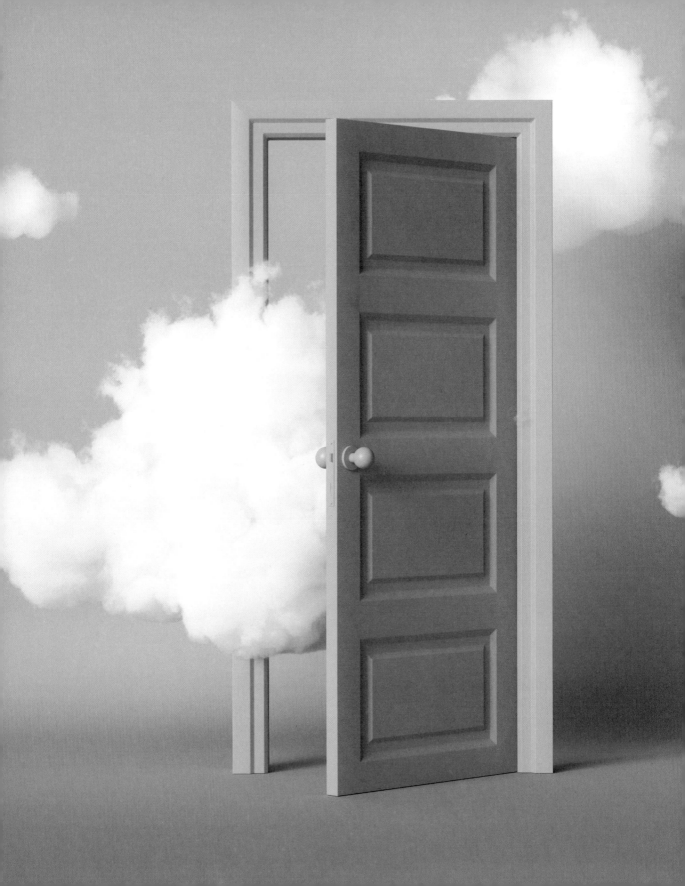

4

WELCOME TO NEVER NEVER LAND

A Guide to Understanding Your Dreams
Through Your Subconscious and Symbolism

*"You may not get everything you
dream about, but you will never get
anything you don't dream about."*

- WILLIAM JAMES -

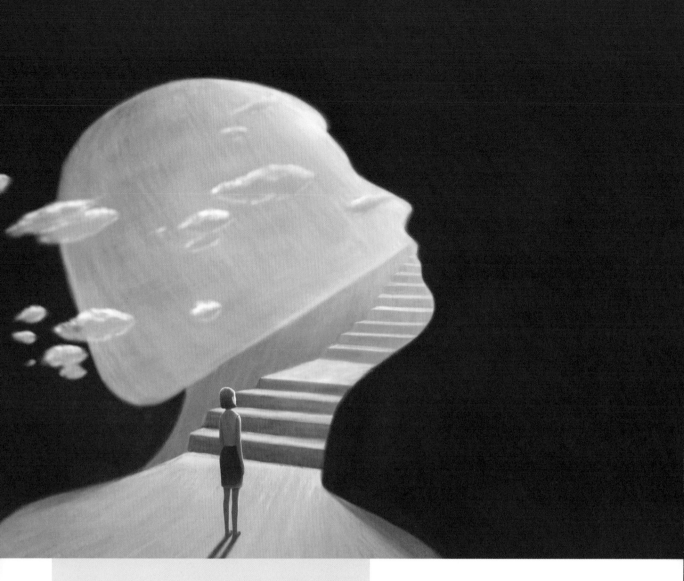

From the outside, sleep looks like a passive activity. The eyes are closed, the body is still, and the breathing is deep. The sleeping individual does not actively interact with their external environment until they wake.

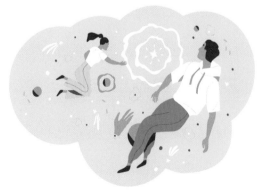

However, on the other side of sleep is the land where dreams exist. This element of sleep is far from passive. Dreams can involve emotional experiences that occur within another fully developed alternate reality. Sometimes we wake and remember them vividly, so vividly that we may feel they were real. Other times we have no recollection of dreaming. We may even be convinced that we didn't dream at all. There are times when we recall our dreams with a kind of mist over our memory, remembering disjointed and confusing bits and pieces of what happened.

————

Due to the very intimate and individual nature of a dream, many elements of dreaming remain a mystery. Some scientists believe dreams are simply the brain's way of sorting through information and processing it. Some psychiatrists believe that dreams allow us to sort through our subconscious emotions and fortify our emotional health. Some mystics believe that dreams contain omens, premonitions, or even warnings. Some spiritualists believe that dreams contain symbols that help guide us in life and serve as a realm to interact with the spirit world.

It is worth exploring your dream life and what you believe it to be—scientific, spiritual, or a combination of the two. This is a worthwhile exploration because dreaming is a large part of your existence. The average person dreams for 90-1twenty minutes a night. That adds up to 730 hours a year. That means that you spend about thirty days, or one month, of each year of your visiting dreamland.

Due to this, it can be beneficial to explore your dream life from different points of view and to pursue different angles until you find a dream interpretation style that resonates with you. This chapter contains a variety of information on dreaming and different ways that you can engage with your dream life to build a more meaningful or connected experience to this mysterious world.

The Science of Dreams

Dreaming is when you experience something similar to waking life—though it may be mythical, fragmented, or fantastic —that occurs while you are asleep. A dream involves visual imagery, but it can also involve your other senses. Some people have dreams full of color, much like the real world, or even color that is more vivid than what is present in daily life. Others dream solely in black and white. A dream is oftentimes also accompanied by very real emotions.

The entire brain is active during your dreams. The visual cortex in your brain, which produces the visual element of your dreams, goes into overdrive while you dream. The amygdala, the part of the brain that is associated with your fear response, is found to be very active while dreaming. Interestingly, the least active parts of the brain while dreaming are the frontal lobes. This area of the brain is responsible for reasonable thought. The low-level of frontal lobe activity might explain why we are able to accept some of the more fantastic or unrealistic elements of dreams while we sleep.

When you wake up and think that you did not dream the night before that is likely untrue; you probably just don't remember the dreams. People who study dreaming believe that the average person has between three and six dreams *every single night*. Each of these dreams is thought to last somewhere between 5 minutes and twenty minutes.

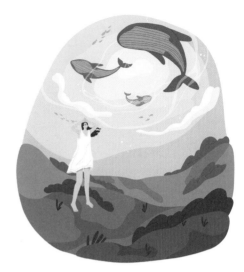

Other Types of Dreams

In addition to the standard dreams that you have, there are also the following types of dreams:

Recurring: a recurring dream is the same dream, similar dream, or same theme recurring over time.

Vivid: a vivid dream is one that feels like it's occurring in real life and everything seems clear.

Lucid: a lucid dream is one in which the dreamer is aware that they are dreaming. Some people claim to be able to control the dream world they inhabit while they are lucid dreaming. If this is true, this could be a valuable skill to safely process emotional and physical experiences in the dream world that may be too fear-inducing in the real world.

Nightmare: a nightmare is a dream that generates strong negative emotions like terror, fear, anxiety, stress, or trauma. The difference between a bad dream and a nightmare is that a nightmare causes you to wake up. Nightmares are hypothesized to be caused by a negative emotional experience or state during the day. Occasionally, nightmares can be caused by medication.

Your Subconscious: The Director of the Movies in Your Mind

The general consensus—though this is still a hypothesis, as dreams are quite a mystery to scientists—is that dreams use experiences and emotions, both those you are conscious of and those that dwell in your subconscious, to create a kind of movie in your mind.

In the scientific world, there are hypothesized benefits of these nightly movies that mainly involve the processing of emotions. Some experts believe that dreams help you file and filter your emotional experiences. Some dream researchers also believe that the function of dreaming is to assist your memory and help it process certain experiences to potentially assist you with solving problems that you are facing in your daily life.

Some of the hypotheses about the purpose dreams serve comes from the information that researchers gethererd about what happens to an individual when to enter the REM sleep stage where the majority of dreaming occurs. When individuals were kept from dreaming, they developed anxiety and depression, had difficulty concentrating, and some experienced hallucinations. This indicates that dreaming is potentially important for emotional regulation, focus, and understanding the difference between illusion and reality.

Setting a Dream Intention

Though dreams are still widely misunderstood, most people studying dreams agree on this: your environment affects your dreams. This involves both your physical environment while asleep and your mental environment prior to sleeping.

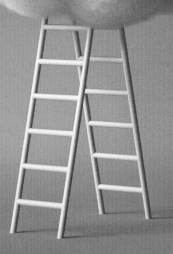

Your Physical Environment

Everything from the food you ate before going to sleep to the smells and sounds around you while you sleep can impact your dreams.

If you eat something that impacts your digestion, it may disrupt your sleep. This can cause you to remember your dreams, but the flipside is that it may also cause you to remember a nightmare, and a nightmare is more likely to occur while you are experiencing a physical disruption like the physical discomfort of digestion. Additionally, if you go to sleep hungry, you might dream about food.

If you hear something while you are asleep, it can make its way into your dreams. This is because our ears still respond to sound while we are asleep as a protective way to alert us to danger in our vulnerable sleep state. If the sounds you are hearing are pleasant, it can help facilitate a pleasant dream. For example, if your roommate puts on classical music you might dream that you are attending a symphony or a luxe party featuring a string-quartet. However, if the sounds you are hearing are chaotic or upsetting, it can trigger a nightmare. For example, if you fall asleep with a movie on in the background and there are gunshots or a loud car crash in the film, you may experience something similar in your dream.

If you smell something, it can also impact the type of dream you have. German researchers made a correlation between things that smell good and positive dreams and things that smell bad and negative dreams. Women who were exposed to the scent of roses while they slept experienced pleasant dreams more frequently than women who were exposed to the scent of rotten eggs while they slept.

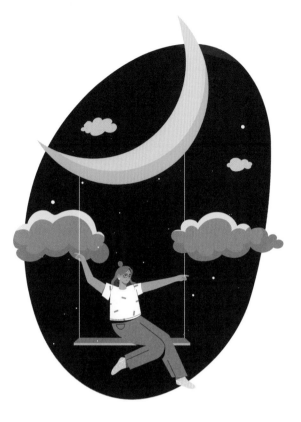

To create an ideal physical environment for dreams:

- Do not eat anything 2-4 hours before bed.

- Block out sound or incorporate sounds that are peaceful or positive

- Utilize calming essential oils on your pillow or in a diffuser to send your brain signals of positivity while you sleep

- Refer to Chapter Two in this book for a fully comprehensive guide to creating an ideal physical environment for sleep and for dreaming

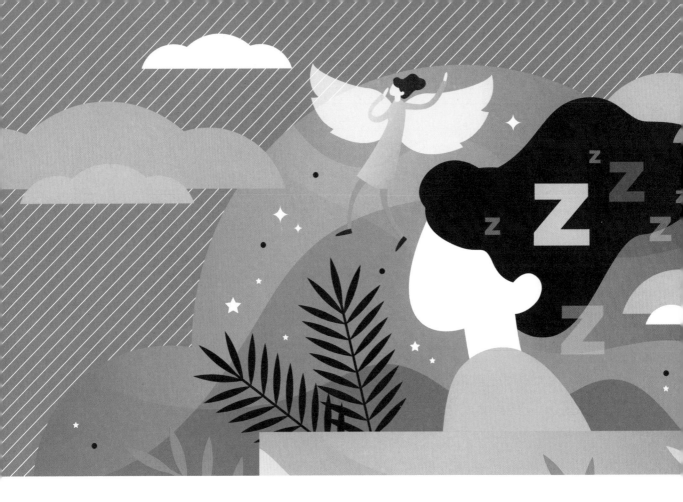

Your Mental Environment

The thoughts that you have prior to going to sleep can impact the dreams you have. If you have racing thoughts, worries, or feel fearful, you will be more prone to having bad dreams or nightmares. You may have to confront the unresolved fear in your dream. If you focus on pleasant thoughts or peaceful imagery before falling asleep, you are more likely to have beautiful dreams.

Repressing a negative thought will not keep it from appearing in a dream and can actually have the opposite effect. When a group of people were asked to repress a negative thought before falling asleep, more people dreamed of that repressed concept than those who were not asked to repress the negative thought.

To create an ideal mental environment for dreams:

- Do not watch any high-anxiety or fear-inducing movies before bed

- Do not play any high-anxiety or fear-inducing video games before bed

- Do not think about what you have to do the next day or anything worrying you

- Set a dream intention

- Refer to Chapter 3 in this book for a fully comprehensive guide to creating an ideal mental environment for sleep and for dreaming

SETTING A DREAM INTENTION

To set a dream intention, simply focus on something you would like to dream about. Make it as wonderful as you can imagine. All you have to do is lie down in bed, close your eyes, and think "I would like to dream about _____."
Fill in the blank with something you desire and include as many details as you can.

DREAM INTENTION EXAMPLES

• I would like to dream about a beautiful vacation. I want to see myself on a beach with a tropical drink in my hand. I want to be able to taste the salt in the air and feel the sand in between my toes. I want to watch the sun dip below the ocean and watch the vibrant colors of the sunset fill the sky.

• I would like to dream about flying. I want to feel myself floating and weightless high above the world. I want to be able to see the treetops and fly above the city lights. I want to end my dream by flying amongst the stars.

• I would like to dream about the perfect world. I want to see everyone smiling and happy and living in harmony. I want to see people hugging and laughing and enjoying one another. I want to walk through the streets of this world and notice all of the beautiful details.

Dream Journals

When deciding whether or not to keep a dream journal, you have to decide if your dream life is important to you. Both scientists and mystics agree that dreams hold information about our emotional processing and help cue us into the general themes we may be dealing with in our lives. If you would like access to this internal information, then a dream journal is for you.

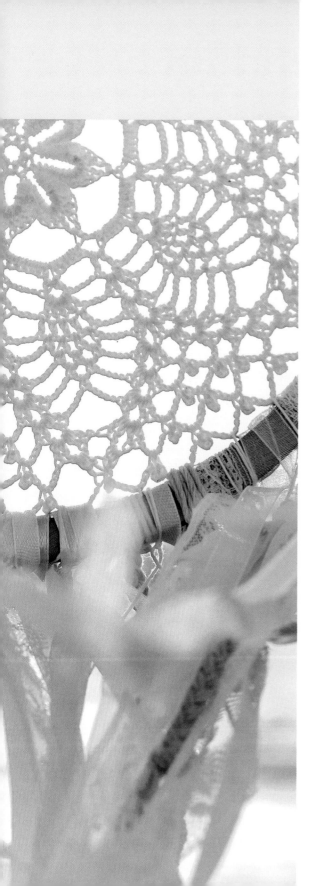

Additionally, many people complain about forgetting their dreams or not remembering them at all. If you fall into this category, you may think that a dream journal would not serve you. The contrary is actually true; committing to a dream journal can help you with dream recall and sharpen your ability to remember your dream life.

—

Keeping a Dream Journal

The concept behind a dream journal is simple. It is a notebook that you keep near your bed. Whenever you wake from a dream, be it in the middle of the night or in the morning, jot down any details you recall in your dream journal. Try to be as specific as possible. Include any emotions you experienced during the dream. You can even include drawings if this helps you.

After jotting down your dream, leave space on the page to write down your interpretations or understanding about your dream—you can use the different schools of thought on dream interpretation below as a guide--—when you revisit your dream during your alert waking hours.

To better facilitate recalling your dreams, you can set an intention before you sleep by stating: *Remembering my dreams is a priority in my life.*

Dream Interpretation

When you are ready to interpret one of the dreams in your dream journal, first find a quiet and comfortable spot for reflection. You can play ambient music if this helps you relax and look within.

The first thing you will do is look at what you wrote about your dream and identify any themes or symbols. Below is a list of common themes and a list of common symbols to help you get started. Remember, your themes/symbols *do not need to be included on these lists.* Anything that you feel is significant in the dream—a person, object, animal, place, emotion, activity, etc. —can classify as a symbol or theme. You can circle these in your dream description or you can list them separately under the dream.

—

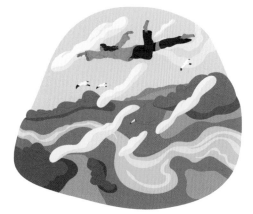

Common Dream Themes

- Being chased
- Being naked
- Being trapped
- Death
- Falling
- Flying
- Inability to speak
- Infidelity
- Losing teeth
- Marriage
- Meeting someone famous
- Missing a flight/being late
- Pregnancy
- Taking a test

Common Dream Symbols

- Animals
- Babies
- Food
- Demons
- Houses
- Money
- Mountains
- People
- Vehicles
- Water

Next, think about any details that stand out or don't seem to make sense. If you don't have anything in this category, don't worry about it. If you do identify some unusual details, note them. They may be sub-themes or sub-symbols or may indicate something else going on in your life or with your emotions.

After identifying the themes, symbols, and significant details, you can begin your process of dream interpretation. The way that you choose to interpret your dreams is entirely up to you. You can go at it alone and utilize your own instinct. This is highly recommended as no one knows your mind better than you do. To interpret your own dream without assistance, think about what the dream, symbols, and themes in it instinctively mean to you. Look deeper into the emotions you were experiencing, and think about what they are trying to tell you about your daily life.

If you need a jumping off point, you can employ one of the schools of thought listed below or use some of their techniques to hone your own dream interpretation skills

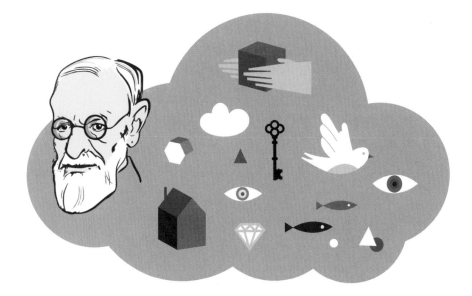

Freud Dream Interpretation

In 1900, Sigmund Freud, a psychologist, published his book The Interpretation of Dreams. Freud believed dreams give you insight into your subconscious fears and desires. More specifically, Freud believed dreams are the "disguised fulfillments of repressed infantile wishes." Due to this, Freud believed that all dreams have meaning.

Freud also believed symbols could not be used as a universal way to interpret dreams. He believed only the individual can interpret their dream. He believed in the idea of free association which is when the individual explores their own feelings and associations with the dream without judgment. Essentially, Freud believed someone can identify the meaning of their dream by identifying different themes, applying those themes to their own life, and figuring out how the dream made them feel.

When using Freud's concept of free association, do not feel the need to connect what you experience in your dream to "repressed infantile wishes" if you feel this is too limiting. Trust yourself to work through free association.

To use your dream journal to practice free association, simply isolate one symbol or theme in your dream and think about it. Figure out what it means to you and write it down.

For example, you may have seen a lion in your dream. You could decide lions are strong and powerful based on the general understanding of a lion. You could also look up what a lion means traditionally in dreams. Freud asks you to do neither of these things. Freud would want you to look at what a lion *means specifically to you*. When you think of a lion, you may think of your favorite stuffed animal when you were little. This stuffed animal was with you from the time you were a baby until your early teens. You had it in your bedroom. Then, one day, the stuffed lion got thrown away. This felt like a violation to you and you did not feel safe without your stuffed lion for months. So, for you, a lion might represent something that provided you safety and then suddenly disappeared. A lion might represent strength to others, but is a symbol of abandonment or grief for you.

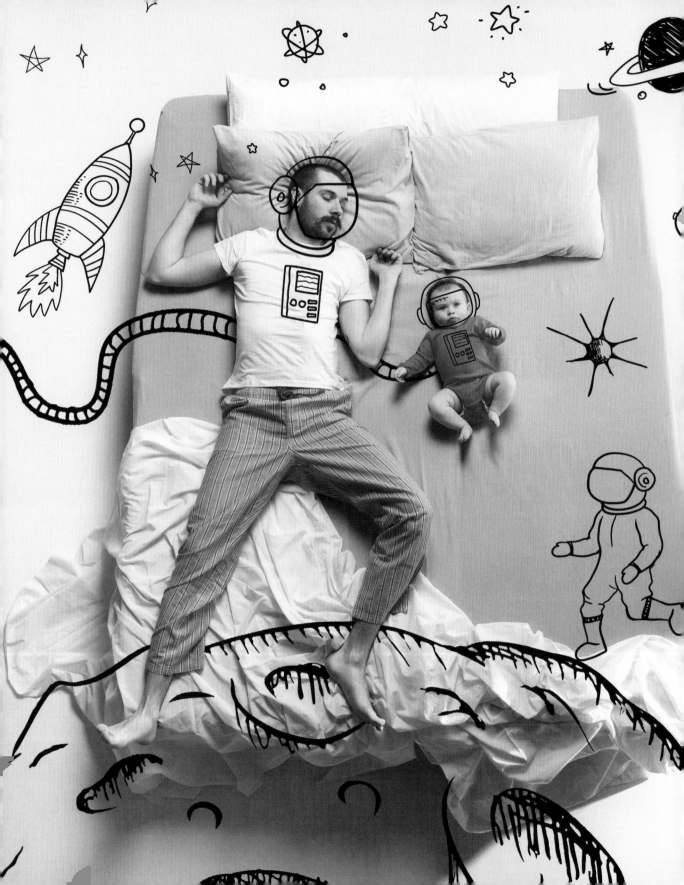

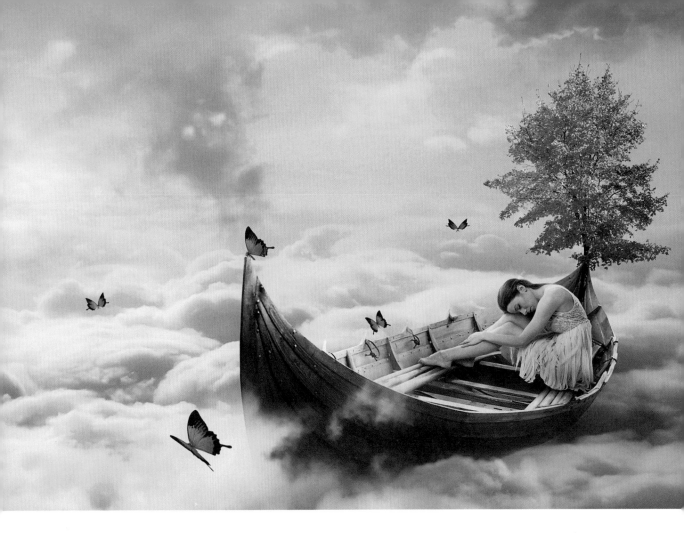

Assisted Dream Interpretation

There are many resources online and in print that can help jumpstart your dream interpretation journey. You can look up the traditional, or commonly held, meaning for many different symbols and themes. There are certain symbols associated with different meanings in the Native American, Shamanic, and Mystic traditions. There are also symbols that have been commonly agreed upon by therapists and dream experts.

If you choose to allow someone else's meaning for a symbol to impact your interpretation, check in with yourself first. Before ascribing to someone else's philosophy, ask yourself a few questions: Does the meaning make sense to you? Does it apply to your life? Is this what your instinct is telling you is correct? If so, feel free to use that as a jumping off point. If not, try to look at the symbol or theme from another perspective.

To give you an idea of what you may uncover on your search, here are some dream themes and symbols with their commonly associated meanings. These are by no means exhaustive and you will likely find different associated meanings on your own dream interpretation journey.

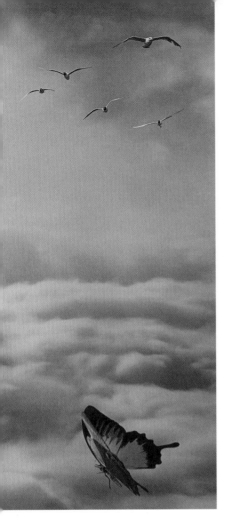

Common Dream Symbols, Themes, and Meanings

Accident: you might be on the wrong track; calling you to assess your current decisions

Attending school: there is a current lesson you need to learn in your life

Baby: that you want a child; that you feel vulnerable; that a blessing is coming your way; that you feel responsible for the people in your life

Being attacked: you do not feel in control of your own life; you are allowing others to tell you what to do

Being late: you feel as if you are running out of time in life; your current life path is incorrect

Boat: if you are on smooth seas, this can indicate that your life is in alignment; if you are on rough waters, it could be an omen of bad luck

Death: you are ready for the current phase of your life to end and for a new one to begin

Falling: you have lost control in your life; you are dealing with anxiety

Flying: a sign of independence and freedom

Ghost: there is an unresolved issue from your past that is haunting your present

Invisible: you feel like you do not get credit for the good things you do in your life

Lost: you are not expressing your true self in daily life; people do not know the "real you"

Talking to an animal: it is time to engage with your creativity; you are craving a deeper connection with nature

Tunnel: self-discovery or internal exploration

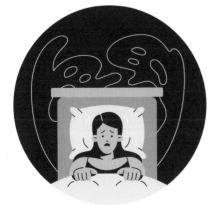

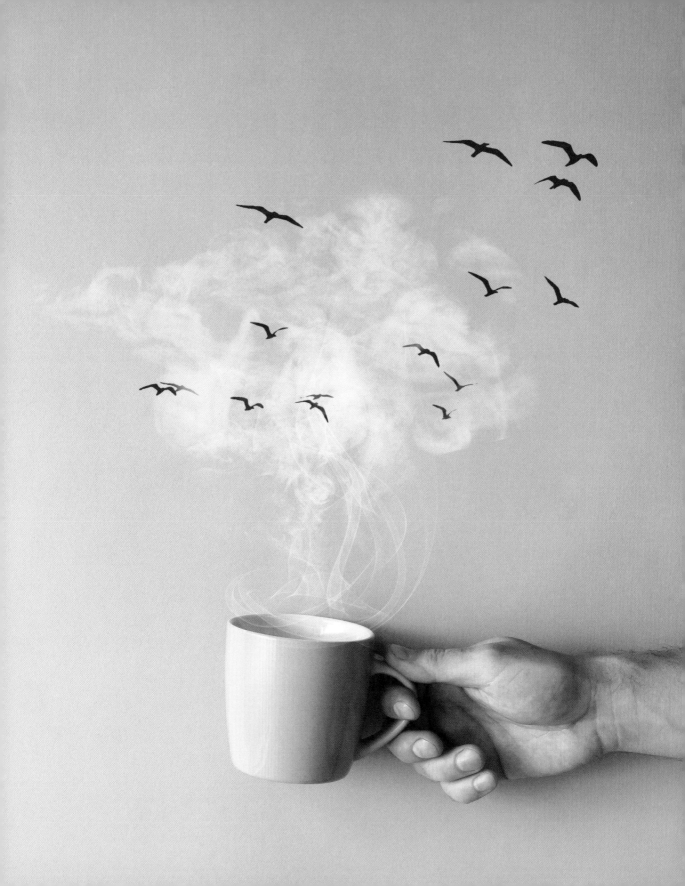

5

RISE AND SHINE WITH INTENTION

How to Wake with Purpose and Thoughtfully
Incorporate Rest Throughout Your Day

"When you rise in the morning,
give thanks for your light,
For your life, for your strength."

- TECUMSEH -

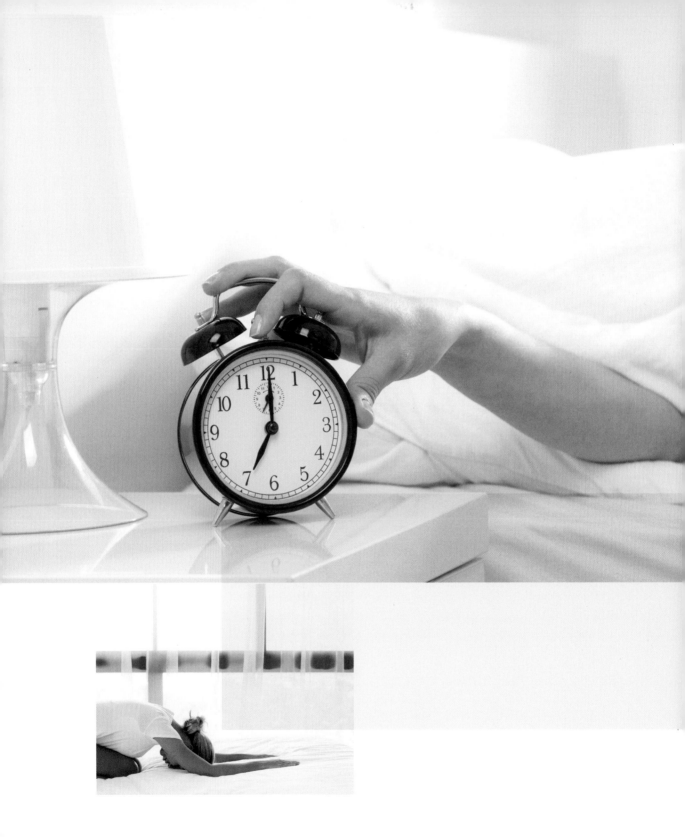

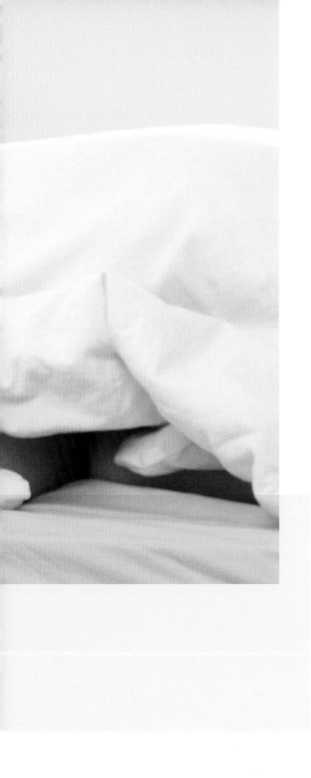

Throughout these pages, you have learned about the importance of sleep. You have been taught tried-and-true strategies to help you sleep more soundly. You have been exposed to things you can incorporate in your life to improve your sleep. And you now know what happens to your mind and body while you sleep. All of this is vital information for you to achieve your optimum sleep health and habits.

If you have fully integrated the lessons in this book, you are likely living the life of a sleep master. You know how to calm yourself for sleep and you prioritize getting quality sleep. You carve out enough time to get your recommended seven-to-nine hours of sleep a night and you wake each morning feeling energized and rested. Now what?

This chapter is all about *what happens after you sleep*. You will benefit from this in a myriad of ways: more control over your moods, increased energy, clearer focus, and a boosted immune system, just to name a few. If you could increase the benefits you get from a good night's sleep by incorporating a few simple habits in the morning, would you?

This section of the book addresses what to do immediately upon waking to extend the benefits of a good night of sleep throughout your whole day. You will learn how to take that extra energy and increased focus and apply it to your life in a thoughtful, intentional, and mindful way. Essentially, sleep is the fuel in your tank. This chapter is about the direction you choose to drive now that you're gassed up.

Let the Light In

The first moments of your day set the tone for the remainder of your day. That means that your waking moments are crucial. The transition from sleeping to waking is also your transition to consciousness. Ideally, you do not want your first moment of consciousness to be full of jarring light, harsh alarm sounds, or the feeling of being rushed. This kind of an environment strips you of some of the sleep benefits—namely feeling centered and present-—you worked so hard to earn.

The good news is that you have control over your waking environment. If you already followed the guidance in Chapter Two, your bedroom will be cued up to be the sleep sanctuary that you need. Have you considered ways that you can make it a waking sanctuary, as well?

—

Determining Your Waking Time

If you have been practicing solid sleep patterns, you are waking up around the same time each day. If you feel rushed in the mornings, you may need to wake up a bit earlier which means that you will have to go to sleep a bit earlier. Factoring in your morning routine and the time it takes to complete everything without feeling rushed is an important consideration. You should have ample time to complete the things you choose or need to do each morning. Your waking time should also incorporate a ten-minute buffer to account for unexpected things that might occur.

Factoring this ten-minute buffer into your morning allows you to get ahead of the things life might throw at you like not being able to find your keys or noticing the pants you were going to wear have a stain on them. This buffer allows you to calmly solve the situation instead of feeling like it interrupted the flow of your day.

Another benefit of the buffer is it allows you time to savor your morning on those days when you don't end up needing to use it. If your morning flows smoothly and you are ready to leave your house yen minutes earlier than usual, soak up those 10 minutes. Slowly sip your cup of coffee. Play a few of your favorite songs and dance before you leave the house. Close your eyes and meditate. Take a short walk. Spend time with your partner or loved ones.

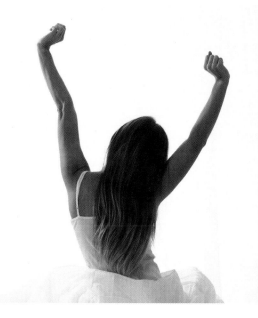

How to Wake Up

Now that you've determined the time you wish to wake up everyday, the next thing to determine is how you would like to wake up. Contrary to popular belief, you do not need to wake up to a loud beeping sound that sharply interrupts your sleep and slams you headfirst into wakefulness.

Learn about different ways you can choose to wake and identify which one sounds appealing to you. Also, feel free to change your waking style to try out the different options.

Natural method

The natural method of waking involves relying on your body's circadian rhythm, which is discussed at length in Chapter One. If you are going to sleep and waking at relatively the same time each day and you are controlling your exposure to unnecessary light in the evening, this method might be the one you prefer.

This method involves going to sleep at your designated bedtime and trusting that your body will wake at the appropriate time after receiving an adequate amount of sleep. This might sound impossible, but you've likely experienced it before. Have you ever woken up a few minutes before the alarm you set is supposed to go off? Or have you ever accidentally forgotten to set your alarm and woken up at the correct time anyway? These things happen because your body's circadian rhythm instinctively knows when to wake.

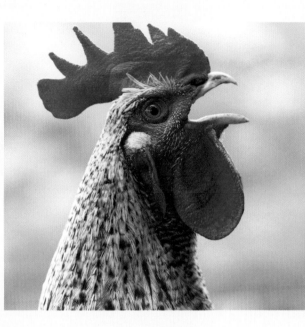

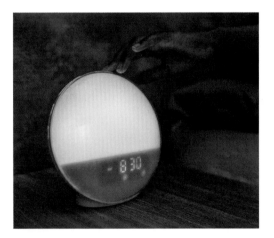

If you feel nervous that you're going to not wake up on time or that you're going to miss something important, set a backup alarm. Once you have established a regular sleeping pattern with predictable sleeping and waking times, your body will begin to know what to do, but the backup alarm can gently assist.

Your backup alarm should be set for thirty minutes after your goal waking time. If your body does not alert you to wake, your alarm will. While you are training your body to wake naturally, add a 30-minute buffer to your morning just in case you have to rely on that backup alarm.

With time and consistency, this is a reliable method for waking and is the easiest way to transition from sleeping to waking because you have allowed your body to transition naturally.

Light method

The light method takes the natural method and gives it some circadian rhythm signaling assistance. Light is one of the key factors that influences your circadian rhythm's sleeping and waking functions. Using light strategically can signal to your brain that it is time to wake up. It is also a smooth transition from sleeping to waking because the gradual increase in light will also allow a gradual transition to waking.

You can influence your circadian rhythm by exposing yourself to light in the morning in a variety of ways.

① **Leave the Blinds Up.** You can leave your blinds up if you live in an area that isn't influenced by artificial external light. For example, if you live in the country, this method might be great for you. However, if you live in the city, your circadian rhythm will be disrupted by the artificial city lights. If you live in an area where you can do this, leave the blinds open so that the sunrise in the morning wakes you up. Note: this can be difficult for some people when the moon is bright, as this keeps some people up. Pay attention to your individual sensitivities.

② **Timer Controlled Blinds.** For those willing to invest in their sleep habits, this option is a great one. There are blinds available that can be controlled by your smartphone and smart home devices. You can assign different times for closing and opening or lowering and raising the blinds. For blinds to be synced with your circadian rhythm, close the blinds completely after sunset. Many of these are also blackout blinds, so you will not have light interrupting your period of sleep. Time the blinds to open about 10 minutes before sunrise. This way, the natural increase in light that occurs during sunrise will assist you in waking.

③ **Light waking device.** For less money than automated blinds, you can purchase a bedside device that uses light to wake you. You set your desired waking time and the device will begin to emit light, first very dim light that gets increasingly brighter light the sunrise, to wake you naturally by your desired time. For those who feel nervous trusting their waking times to light and light alone, this is a good option because most of these devices have a backup alarm that sounds if the light does not wake you.

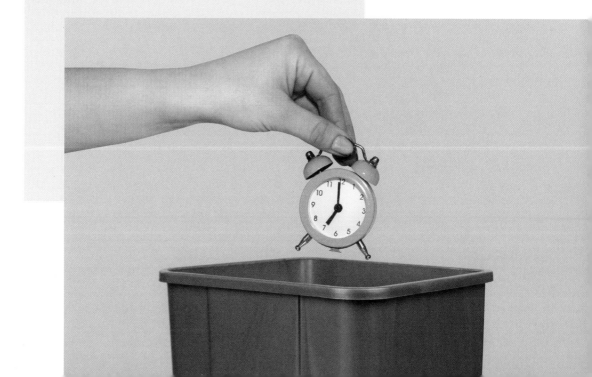

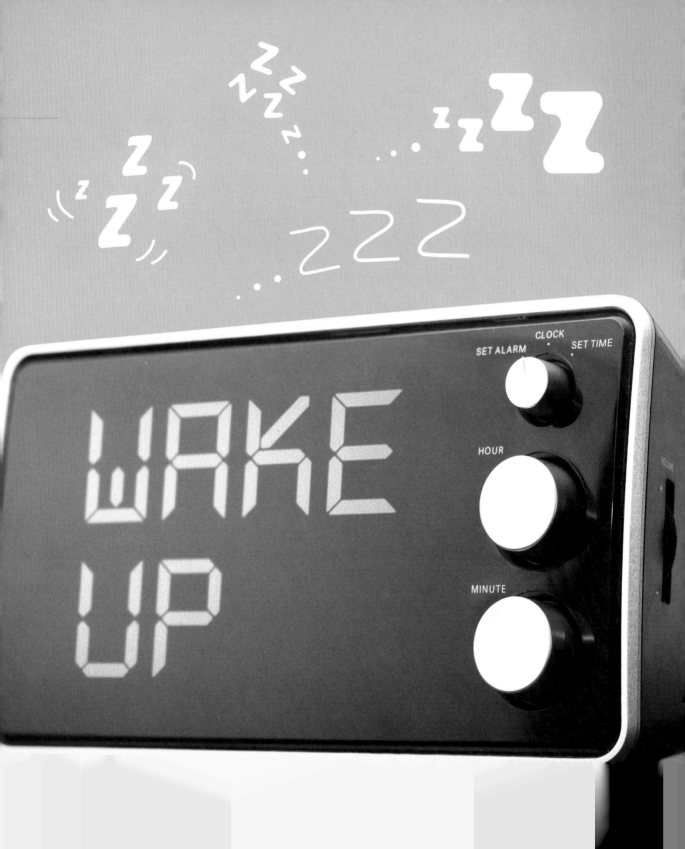

Alarm method

If you are one of countless people who choose to wake using an alarm, let's look at ways that you can optimize your waking method.

Think about the style of alarm you are using. If you are using an old fashioned alarm that uses a beeping sound or radio music to wake you, throw it out. There is nothing natural, gentle, or soothing about a loud robotic beeping noise or the static of a radio station.

If you are using your cell phone, that's another thing that isn't serving you. Keeping your cell phone in your bedroom exposes you to blue light, it emits harmful radiation that is typically near your head as you sleep, and many of the sounds included on the phone as alarm choices are not pleasant noises in the morning, or ever. If you must keep your cell phone in the bedroom and use it as an alarm, place it on the other side of the room. This way, you are not as close to the harmful radiation or blue light and you will have to walk across the room to wake up. Also, upgrade your alarm sound. Download an app with alarm sounds that are pleasing, like ambient music or nature sounds.

If you would like to use an alarm to wake, try investing in a bedside alarm clock made specifically for gentle waking. There are many alarm clocks on the market with a large library of waking sounds and even clocks that take into account different kinds of waking. For example, you might be someone who likes to wake up and still lie in bed for a few minutes. You might want an alarm clock that allows you to set two separate alarms, the first with a very gentle sound and the second with a slightly more impactful sound to get you out of bed. Some of these alarm clocks even have sleep sounds and guided meditations and breathwork practices on them for an added nighttime benefit. Additionally, many of today's alarm clocks have a blackout mode that allows you to stop all light emitting from the device while you sleep.

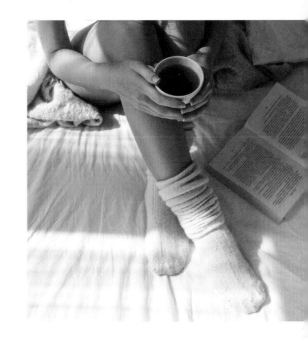

The Power of the Slow Start

Once you have woken up, do not feel the need to jump out of bed. Allow the sleep you just experienced to really sink in. Feel free to stretch and move a bit before you get out of bed.

Once you are ready to leave your bed, you can continue to enjoy the last remnants of your sleep by extending the cozy feeling. You can designate a zone near your bed to store some comfortable items that you can put on first thing. Invest in some comfortable slippers and a robe for yourself. Your robe can be flannel for extra warmth, cotton for ease and breathability, or something like silk or satin for a luxurious start to your day. Keeping yourself cozy allows you to continue to wake up gradually as your circadian rhythm begins to release cortisol to assist you with waking fully.

Once you have covered your feet in your slippers and wrapped your body in your robe, you can begin your morning routine. You will create this routine in the next section.

Your Morning Routine

If you create a routine, or ritual, for your morning, you can stretch your sleep benefits even further. A routine is, by definition, something predictable. This predictability allows your brain to relax, as it does not need to engage in any critical thinking. The presence of a morning routine allows your brain to wake slowly and naturally.

Wake with Water

Water is a wonderful element to incorporate into your morning ritual to signal to your body that it's time to engage with the day.

If you are not someone who likes to shower first thing in the morning, you can still use water in your routine. Go to your sink and run some cold water. Splash it on your face a few times. Gently pat your face dry.

If you are someone who enjoys a morning shower to start the day, there are two types of showers you can try. These two types of showers can also be combined.

Cold Shower

If you are new to cold showers, give yourself time to acclimate to the idea. You can take a normal shower and finish off with a short burst of cold water as you are getting started. Work up to thirty seconds. Then work up to a minute. Eventually, get yourself to the point where you can endure—and even enjoy!—a two-to-three minutes cold shower.

Once you are at the point where you are ready to start your day with a cold shower—and no warm water to ease into it—you can let your body adjust by first running your hands and feet under the water and then taking a few deep breaths before stepping in. Do not hold your breath during the shower. Instead, breathe deeply, allowing the oxygen in your lungs and the cool water on your skin to energize you.

Cold showers have many health benefits. Starting your day with a cold shower makes you alert and helps you feel fresh and awake. It also boosts your immune system, decreases stress, and aids in weight loss. There are added beauty benefits to cold showers—they are less drying than hot showers, so your hair and skin will appear healthier and more hydrated. Additionally, cold showers have been shown to reduce the symptoms of depression.

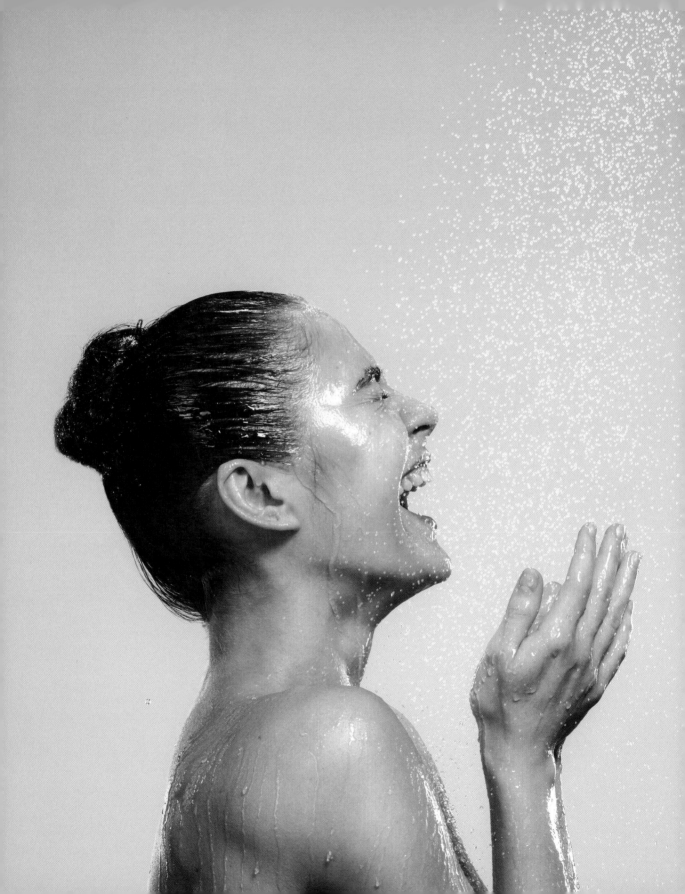

Invigorating Shower

If a cold shower isn't for you, or if you choose to start with a warm shower and then finish with a cold shower, then you will enjoy an invigorating shower specifically designed for the morning hours.

(1) **Dry brush your body.** Before you get into the shower, exfoliate your skin and get your circulation working. To exfoliate your skin, use a method called dry brushing. Use a natural bristled brush with firm bristles. Start at your feet and work your way up using long strokes or circular strokes. Dry brushing should never hurt. If you feel any pain, lighten the pressure you are using or stop. This form of body brushing helps to remove dead skin cells and makes the skin smoother, plumper, and healthier. It also aids in the release of toxins.

(1) **Utilize invigorating products with aromatherapy benefits.** If you are using products like body wash, shaving cream, shampoo, and conditioner, consider purchasing some products that are specific to your morning routine. Think of scents that you find invigorating and fresh: citrus, mint, and bright florals all work. If you would like to make your own scent, you can purchase unscented products and give them a boost with some of your favorite brightly scented essential oils. You can also soak a sponge in eucalyptus or lemon oil and place it in your shower for added aromatherapy benefits.

(1) **Use a scalp massager when washing or rinsing your hair.** Consider incorporating a silicone scalp massager into your morning shower. This affordable product helps promote circulation on the head and scalp, allows products to penetrate more deeply, decreases dandruff, and can promote hair growth. After you apply shampoo to your hair, hold the scalp brush in your hand and use it to help work the shampoo into a lather and exfoliate your scalp. Rub the scalp massager in circular motions all around your head. If you are using a refreshing or minty shampoo, you may experience an increased tingly sensation. As an added bonus, this device increases the pleasure of your shampoo experience - you get clean hair and a head massage at the same time.

(1) **Visualize yourself enjoying your day.** Your morning shower is a great time to begin to focus on your mindset for the day ahead. Smile while you shower. Studies have shown that smiling—even if it feels forced—helps release endorphins, or happy hormones, in the brain. Think about how centered, calm, focused, and kind you'll be throughout the day. Say aloud, "I am looking forward to all of the experiences I will have on this beautiful day."

(1) **Lock in your shower benefits with body oil.** As soon as you turn the water off, pat your body dry with a towel. Patting the skin is gentle on it and also does not remove all of the moisture. While your skin is slightly damp, lock in the moisture with body oil. You can choose a body oil with a scent you love (and now you can skip the perfume!) or you can make your own with a combination of oils and essential oils.

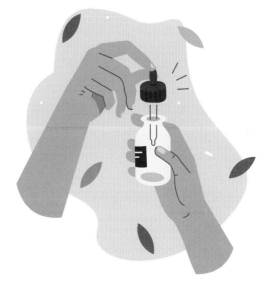

Start with Self-Care

Create Your Own Wake-Up Ritual

Much like the bedtime ritual you created in Chapter Three, you will be creating a morning ritual that helps you wake-up with a positive and focused mindset.

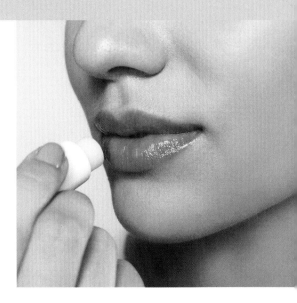

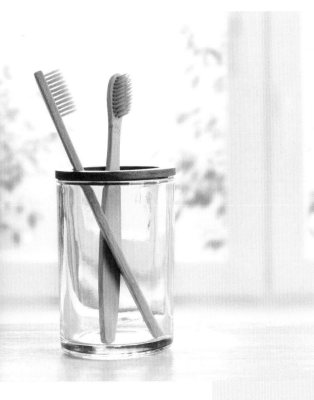

BRUSHING YOUR TEETH/ORAL CARE

Brushing Your Teeth: if you followed the guidance in Chapter Three, you likely already upgraded your toothbrush and have identified a nighttime toothpaste. Have you thought about your morning toothpaste? You should choose something that is flavored in a way that energizes you and makes you feel fresh. Perhaps you would like a spearmint or peppermint flavored toothpaste for fresh breath. Maybe you like the cheerful taste of citrus; you can try an orange or herbal citrus toothpaste.

Tongue Scraper: after a long, restful night of sleep, your mouth might need some extra love to help fight bad breath. Consider using a tongue scraper in the morning to get rid of breath busting bacteria.

SKINCARE AND FACIAL MASSAGE

Cleansing Your Skin: if you went to sleep after completing your nighttime skin routine, all you have to do is splash your face with cold water. If you slept with an overnight treatment or mask on your face, you may need to first remove this with a washcloth and warm water and then finish by splashing cold water on your face.

Skin treatments: daytime skin treatments usually focus on making the under eyes look bright, fresh, rested, and hydrated. Look for a light under eye gel or oil that works with your skin type. You may also want to use a vitamin C treatment to increase brightness, decrease discoloration, and fight aging.

Moisturizing: consider using a moisturizer with SPF included. If you start your day by protecting your delicate facial skin from the sun, you won't have to think about it for the rest of the day. Sun protection is a key component of keeping skin youthful, healthy, and cancer-free.

Lip treatment: choose a hydrating formula with SPF. You can choose something minty to give an extra boost to your morning. The skin on the lips is often forgotten when applying sunscreen and this is why many people show signs of aging on and around their mouth.

Ice Rolling: after you let your moisturizer sink in for a couple of minutes, utilize an ice roller to help the product absorb more deeply, decrease puffiness, and help drain toxins from your face. Ice rolling is exactly what it sounds like. A rolling device with a frozen component is used to rub all over your face. The icy feeling helps to wake you up, while it removes some of the fluid retention that causes a puffy face. You can take your time rolling the icy tool across parts of your face that might need a little extra love, like swollen eyes or a sore jaw. Spend anywhere from five to fifteen minutes rolling your face. You can listen to spa-like music to further enhance your experience.

HAIRCARE

Hairbrush: if your hair is wet from the shower, use a wet brush or a wide toothed comb to work through any tangles without damaging your hair.

Leave-In Conditioner: if your hair is still damp from your shower, think about applying a leave-in conditioner to treat your hair and to let it air dry, at least most of the way. The less heat you use on your hair, the better its condition will be. Also, using a hair dryer can be a very loud, hot, and disruptive start to the morning. If you want to go the completely air-dried route, you can find products that are specifically formulated for making your air-dried hair look the best it can. There are countless styling balms, sprays, foams, and creams that can make your hair dry faster, combat frizz, promote curls, or lock in shine.

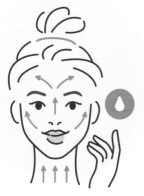

Take a Rest Assessment

As the final step in your rise-and-shine routine, ask yourself, "Do I feel rested?" Answer honestly. If you do feel rested, reflect on what is working for you in regards to your sleep health and habits. If you do not feel rested, reflect on what you would like to change or implement to improve upon your sleep quality.

The Big Four

After you have gotten up and shown yourself a good amount of self-care, you can move onto the Big Four, or the foundational building blocks for your mindset that day. The idea behind the Big Four is that once you complete these four tasks, you are in control of your day, not the other way around. Strategically setting aside time to fortify your mindset not only helps you become more positive, it also helps you manage your levels of stress and anxiety during the day which will result in you achieving better sleep at night.

To give yourself enough time to complete the Big Four in the morning, block out thirty-five minutes. During these this time, you will complete your daily Affirmation, Hydration, Movement, and Gratitude practices.

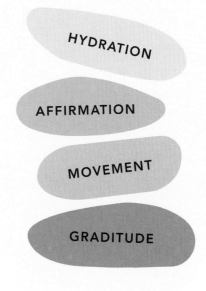

HYDRATION

AFFIRMATION

MOVEMENT

GRADITUDE

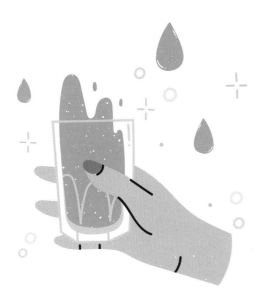

Hydration - 3 Minutes

Take three minutes to slowly sip a full glass of water in the morning. Your body dehydrates while you sleep and it needs water for many of its essential functions. Water strengthens the immune system, helps with clear thinking and focus, assists with maintaining a healthy weight, flushes toxins, and increases the beauty of the skin and hair. If you want to drink a glass of water that has added health benefits and helps start your day off with its bright flavors, you can add the juice of a lemon and some fresh mint to your morning glass.

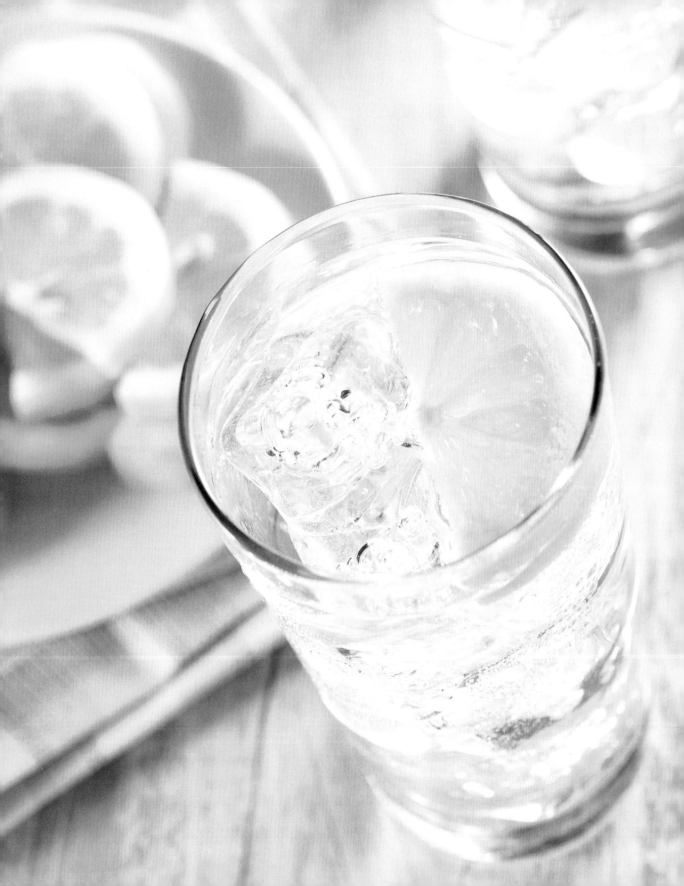

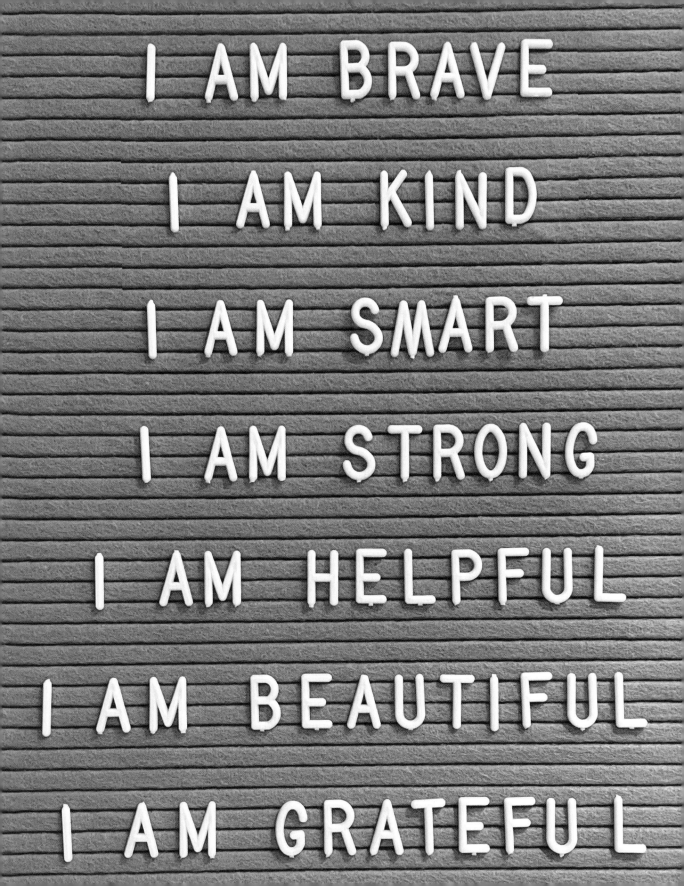

Affirmation - 2 Minutes

An affirmation is a positive thought or statement, written or spoken, that challenges self-limiting beliefs and replaces patterns of negative thinking with patterns of positive thinking. An affirmation can be spoken, written down, looked at, or listened to. The affirmation practice that you are going to create involves all of these things and is short, simple, and easy to incorporate into your morning.

① **Grab a Post-it note and a pen.** Sit down—you can continue to sip your water while you do this if you have not yet finished it—and prepare to write your affirmation.

② **Briefly think about yourself and your day and identify an obstacle.** Whatever "obstacle" you identify is going to be removed through the use of your affirmation.

③ **Negate the obstacle with an affirmation.** If the obstacle is feeling like you don't have enough time in the day, your affirmation will state the opposite. You could write down something like "I am excellent at time management," or "I have all the time I need."

If the obstacle is a personal insecurity, like feeling like you are too shy to accomplish what you want, knock it down with your affirmation. You could write down something like "I speak my mind" or "The right words come to me easily and I speak them with confidence."

If you cannot think of an affirmation for the day, feel free to borrow one of these:

- I trust myself to make the right decisions for my life.
- I have a good heart, and I am a wonderful person.
- I have the tools to navigate any circumstance I might encounter.
- I am brilliant and creative, and I inspire myself and others.
- I am absolutely beautiful and perfectly made.
- I am a great cook and make the best chocolate chip cookies ever.
- I have a wonderful sense of humor, and people enjoy being around me.
- I am an asset to the workplace and to my co-workers.

④ **Write your chosen affirmation on your Post-it note.** Speak it aloud with conviction three times. Hear yourself say it. Stick the Post-it note somewhere you will see it throughout the day: on your fridge, on a mirror, on your phone, in your car, wherever.

⑤ **Read it throughout the day to remind yourself of how capable you truly are.**

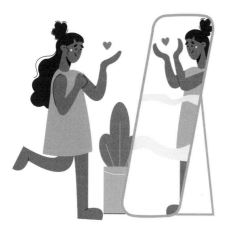

Movement - thirty minutes

Right after you finish your affirmation exercise, get moving. This signals to your body that your day has officially begun and you are ready for action, while also allowing you some responsibility-free time to give your brain time to catch up. Also, exercise helps lift your mood which carries through to the rest of your day.

If you live somewhere that weather allows, get outside for a morning walk. This is a great way to complete your recommended thirty minutes of daily exercise at the beginning of the day, breathe fresh air deeply into your lungs, and get a dose of mood and immune system boosting vitamin D. For additional mood-boosting benefits, listen to some of your favorite uplifting or inspiring music during your walk. Avoid listening to anything combative or talk-radio oriented during this time, as this can unwittingly trigger stress responses.

If you live somewhere with inclement weather, you can still move inside. You can utilize a treadmill or stationary bike, engage in a gentle yoga flow, or turn on your music and dance. Any kind of movement that you choose to engage in is beneficial.

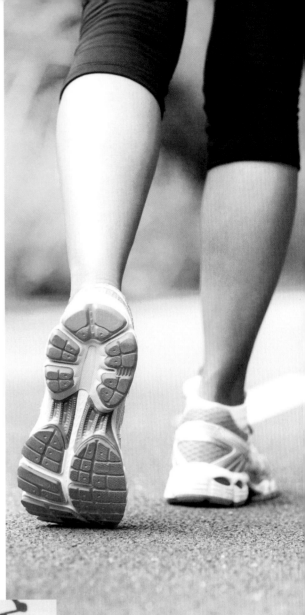

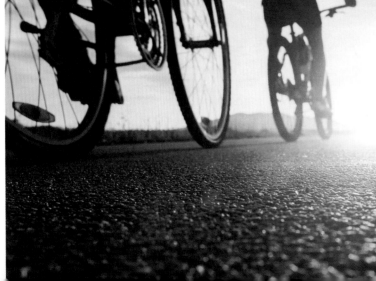

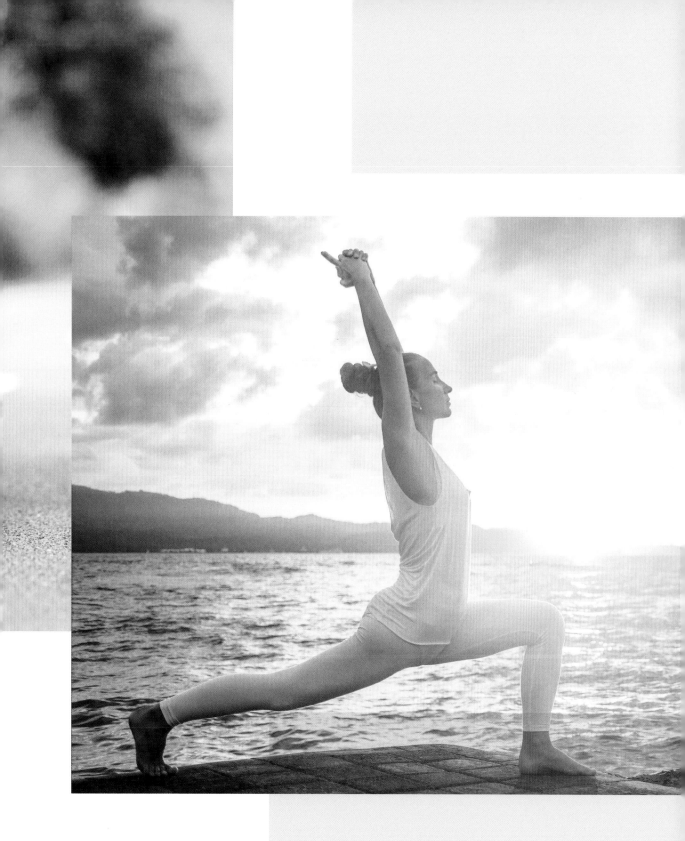

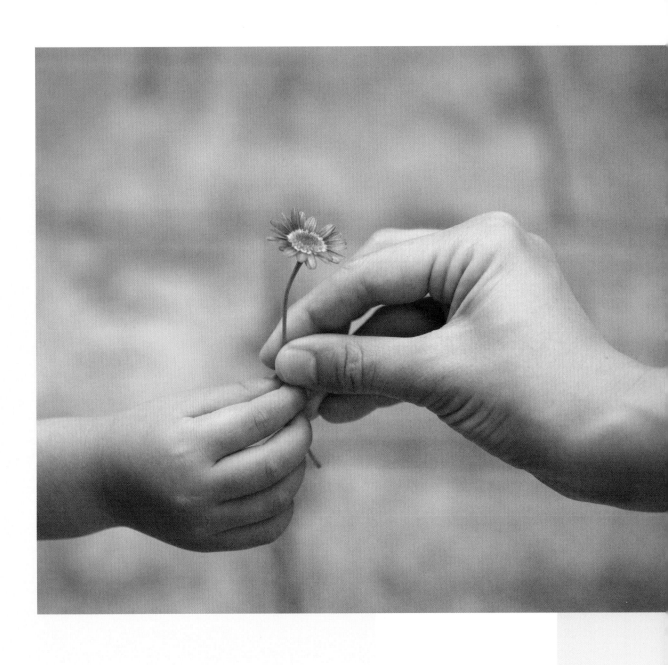

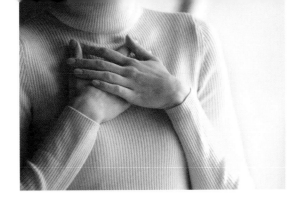

Give Gratitude

You will hone in on gratitude concurrently with your thirty minutes of movement. At the ten minute, twenty minute, and thirty minute mark of your morning movement, ask yourself, "What am I grateful for?" This can be anything. It can be a person, an experience, a memory, a quality, a dream, something practical, or something totally impractical. Force yourself to answer the question in your mind in detail. Elaborate to yourself as to why you are grateful for what you chose. Exploring the reason for your gratitude helps you more fully connect to it and understand it. Additionally, the more time you spend in a state or gratitude, the less room there is for negativity to enter your mind.

For example: instead of saying that you are grateful for your husband, you would think about all the reasons why you are grateful for him. Maybe you're grateful that he says you're beautiful. Perhaps you're grateful that he kisses you each morning before work. Maybe you're grateful that someone else understands your obsession with stand up comedy and historical fiction. Maybe you're so happy that you have someone to watch movies with. It doesn't matter how strange the reason may seem, seek it. Seek all the reasons. You will likely find that stating who or what you're grateful for is the tip of the gratitude iceberg. All the incredible reasons why you are experiencing a feeling of thanks are the real substance of the gratitude iceberg hiding just below the surface.

Incorporating Mindfulness

When you step out into the day after a restful night of sleep and after completing your uplifting morning routine, the rest of your day will be absolutely perfect and run without a hitch.

Don't you wish it was that easy?

—

Likely, at some point during the day, something will not go your way. Maybe you'll forget that you had a dentist appointment or you double-booked your lunch. Maybe you'll get a flat tire or the school parking attendant flips you the bird. Maybe your coffee order is wrong or you got passed over for the promotion that you wanted.

All of these things have the potential to completely derail your day. The secret is this: they only have the power to do that if you give them that power.

You have a choice, and that choice is in how you react. The next time you feel like all the hard work that you put in to get your mindset right is about to go down the drain, try one of the following three exercises to get yourself back into alignment.

Stop and Breathe

Any time you experience overwhelm, stress, anger, hopelessness, or negativity that shifts your mindset to a bad place, you can quickly reset this by using your breath.

Stop where you are and place one hand over your belly and the other over your heart. Close your eyes and say, "I exhale negativity. I inhale positivity."

Breathe deeply through your nose, down into your belly, and out through your mouth ten times. At the end, open your eyes and shake out your arms and legs.

If you don't feel any more at peace than you did before beginning or you would like to release even more negativity, repeat the exercise.

5-Minute Anxiety Release

Go somewhere where you can have five minutes of privacy and peace. Identify your anxiety. Write it down. You can do this on your smartphone or on a piece of paper. Write down everything that you can identify that is making you feel anxious. Now, write at the end, "The anxiety I am feeling does not serve me. It is not mine to feel. I release it." Then cross out or delete everything you wrote that made you feel anxious. Now you are only left with what you wrote at the end. Speak it aloud and exhale forcefully afterward.

Visualization to get Present

When the world around you feels chaotic and out of control, you can find solace in the fact that you have all the tools you need to create an environment of peace in your mind.

Find somewhere you can sit alone for ten minutes. If you do not have the luxury of taking ten minutes away, even a minute or two of this visualization exercise can have benefits.

Sit comfortably, close your eyes, and breathe slowly. Imagine yourself in a beautiful green meadow surrounded by yellow flowers. It is a warm day and you can feel the sun hit your skin. This sensation is only interrupted by a cool breeze. There is a beautiful stream at the edge of the meadow with clear flowing water. Allow yourself to explore this visualization. Imagine yourself exploring this environment and interacting with your surroundings. Feel free to add any beautiful elements that you choose.

At the end of your visualization, open your eyes. Say, "I carry this peaceful world within me wherever I go."

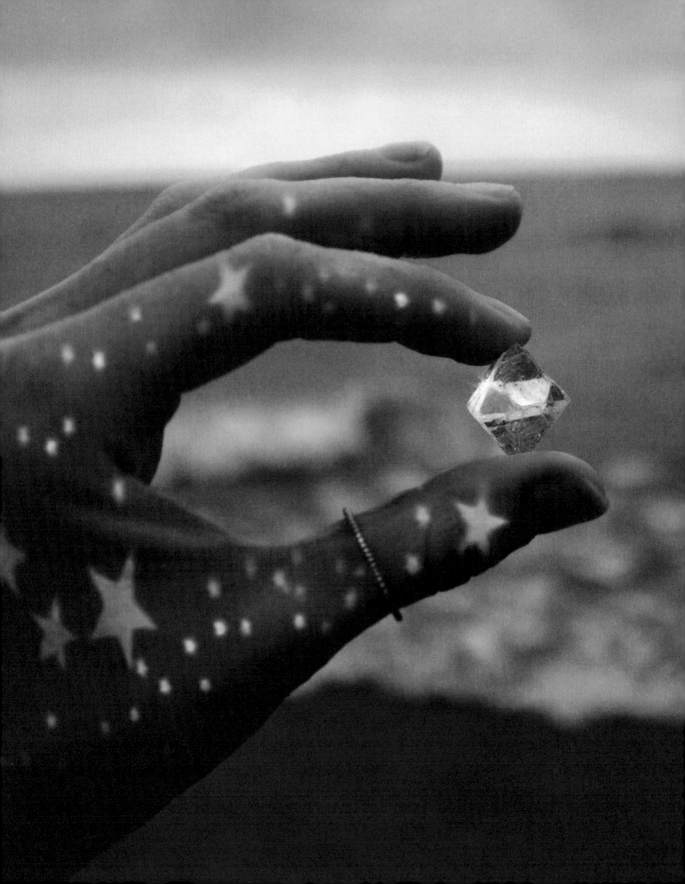

Stay in Touch

I feel strongly about being part of a community
that's committed to self-care and supports and
encourages one another along the self-care
journey—and I'd love to stay in contact with you!

If you'd like to connect with me,
you can find me on Instagram:

@blonderambitions

If this book resonated with you,
I would be honored if you would share it
on social media! Please use the hashtag:

#thecompleteguidetoselfcare

I have an extensive background in speaking
at conventions, symposiums, retreats, workshops,
on podcasts, and online. If you'd like to book
a speaking engagement, please email me at:

blonderambitions.kiki@gmail.com

Thank You & Acknowledgments

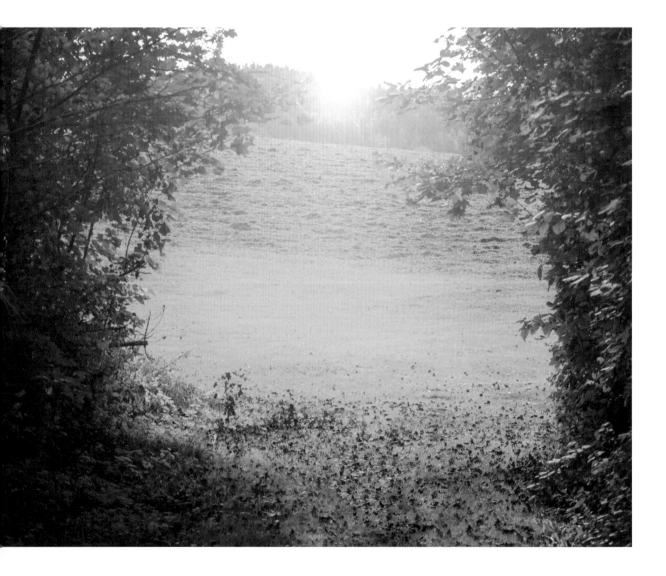

This book would not have been possible without my mother and my brother—two of the greatest loves of my life. The days got considerably dimmer and the nights even darker when their souls left this physical plane. After losing them, I began to walk the long path of grief—a path that impacted not just my waking moments, but the moments when I unsuccessfully attempted to find escape in the realm of sleep. It has been a long and trying journey to learn to sleep again, but I have arrived. And I am so grateful to have an opportunity to share what I have learned with you.

Words in this book that feel like a reassuring warm hug, a dose of self-belief, or like you are being tucked in at night would not have been possible without the love of my mother—an earth angel in life and a true angel after her transition.

Words that help you understand the mechanics of sleep, the body, or the brain would not have been possible without the conversations I so dearly miss having with my brother - a brilliant mind who sought to learn and teach the connection of the brain, the body, and the spirit.

I am endlessly grateful to my father for his unwavering belief in me and for exposing me to the power and the beauty of the written word. Some of my fondest childhood memories are of looking through his extensive collection of books, the treasures of a self-taught man. Another lovely memory I have is frequently knocking softly on the door to my father's study while he wrote to ask if he could take a quick break to read me something from his latest book. I remember feeling so valued when he not only took the time to read to me, but to also ask my nine-year-old opinion of what he had written. I am so grateful to have his footsteps to guide me as I, too, take the writer's path.

Many authors report that they feel alone in their journey. I do not. I am grateful beyond words to have the gift of the constant love and support of my sister, my very first friend and my best friend to this day. Meeting her is like being in the room with the sun. She is made of light and makes life feel like summer. A large source of inspiration in writing this book is her: a sleep-deprived supermom of two young children who are her source of endless joy and unutterable exhaustion. I often find it easiest to write when I imagine the person I am serving with my writing. I, of course, did my best to imagine each of you. I also constantly thought of ways to make my sister's life easier. I thought of what practical tips would help her sleep in her current chaotically wonderful situation.

My heart, which is still in the process of healing after an earth-shattering loss, would not have been in the state it needed to be to write this book without my husband. I am eternally grateful for the smart man with the kindest eyes who taught me to laugh again. I did not think I would ever get married, but I also did not think that I would ever meet an earnest conversationalist who traded ego for the much more interesting path of humble curiosity. His goodness inspires me every single day. I'm so glad I married him three months before the completion of this book. It's the best decision I've made to date.

I give thanks to God. The greatest source of love, life, and hope. My guiding light that is interwoven in every facet of my life. The source of dreams. Thank you for the beautiful mystery you have gifted all of us.

Finally, to each of you. For taking the time to care for yourself. For acknowledging the rest that you so deeply deserve. For raising the vibration of this place we currently inhabit.

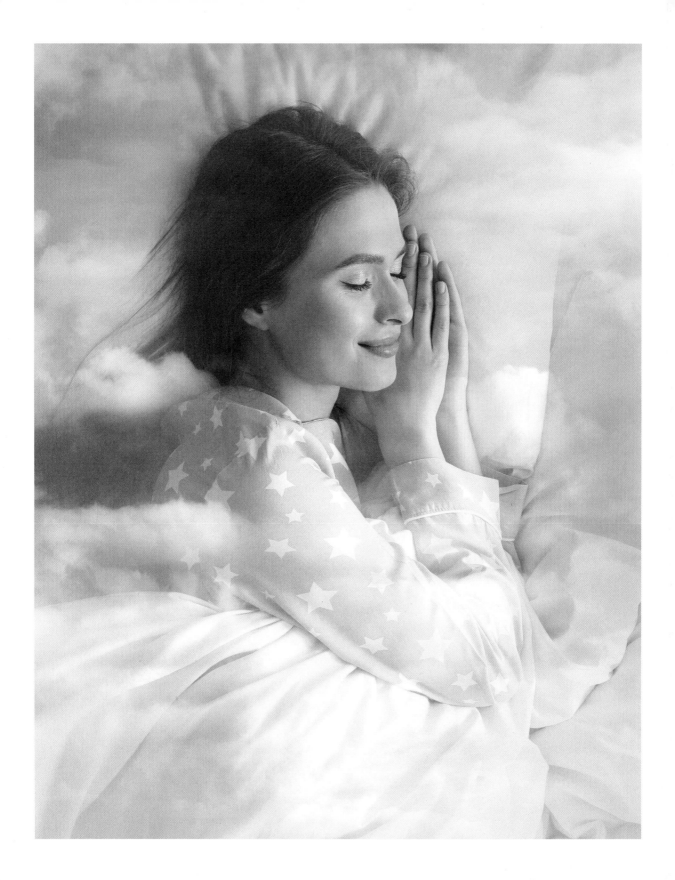